ATS-19 ADMISSION TEST SERIES

This is your
PASSBOOK for...

RN

Nursing School Entrance Examinations for Registered and Graduate Nurses

Test Preparation Study Guide
Questions & Answers

NATIONAL LEARNING CORPORATION®

COPYRIGHT NOTICE

This book is SOLELY intended for, is sold ONLY to, and its use is RESTRICTED to individual, bona fide applicants or candidates who qualify by virtue of having seriously filed applications for appropriate license, certificate, professional and/or promotional advancement, higher school matriculation, scholarship, or other legitimate requirements of education and/or governmental authorities.

This book is NOT intended for use, class instruction, tutoring, training, duplication, copying, reprinting, excerption, or adaptation, etc., by:

1) Other publishers
2) Proprietors and/or Instructors of "Coaching" and/or Preparatory Courses
3) Personnel and/or Training Divisions of commercial, industrial, and governmental organizations
4) Schools, colleges, or universities and/or their departments and staffs, including teachers and other personnel
5) Testing Agencies or Bureaus
6) Study groups which seek by the purchase of a single volume to copy and/or duplicate and/or adapt this material for use by the group as a whole without having purchased individual volumes for each of the members of the group
7) Et al.

Such persons would be in violation of appropriate Federal and State statutes.

PROVISION OF LICENSING AGREEMENTS – Recognized educational, commercial, industrial, and governmental institutions and organizations, and others legitimately engaged in educational pursuits, including training, testing, and measurement activities, may address request for a licensing agreement to the copyright owners, who will determine whether, and under what conditions, including fees and charges, the materials in this book may be used them. In other words, a licensing facility exists for the legitimate use of the material in this book on other than an individual basis. However, it is asseverated and affirmed here that the material in this book CANNOT be used without the receipt of the express permission of such a licensing agreement from the Publishers. Inquiries re licensing should be addressed to the company, attention rights and permissions department.

All rights reserved, including the right of reproduction in whole or in part, in any form or by any means, electronic or mechanical, including photocopying, recording, or by any information storage and retrieval system, without permission in writing from the Publisher.

Copyright © 2025 by
National Learning Corporation

212 Michael Drive, Syosset, NY 11791
(516) 921-8888 • www.passbooks.com
E-mail: info@passbooks.com

PASSBOOK® SERIES

THE *PASSBOOK® SERIES* has been created to prepare applicants and candidates for the ultimate academic battlefield – the examination room.

At some time in our lives, each and every one of us may be required to take an examination – for validation, matriculation, admission, qualification, registration, certification, or licensure.

Based on the assumption that every applicant or candidate has met the basic formal educational standards, has taken the required number of courses, and read the necessary texts, the *PASSBOOK® SERIES* furnishes the one special preparation which may assure passing with confidence, instead of failing with insecurity. Examination questions – together with answers – are furnished as the basic vehicle for study so that the mysteries of the examination and its compounding difficulties may be eliminated or diminished by a sure method.

This book is meant to help you pass your examination provided that you qualify and are serious in your objective.

The entire field is reviewed through the huge store of content information which is succinctly presented through a provocative and challenging approach – the question-and-answer method.

A climate of success is established by furnishing the correct answers at the end of each test.

You soon learn to recognize types of questions, forms of questions, and patterns of questioning. You may even begin to anticipate expected outcomes.

You perceive that many questions are repeated or adapted so that you can gain acute insights, which may enable you to score many sure points.

You learn how to confront new questions, or types of questions, and to attack them confidently and work out the correct answers.

You note objectives and emphases, and recognize pitfalls and dangers, so that you may make positive educational adjustments.

Moreover, you are kept fully informed in relation to new concepts, methods, practices, and directions in the field.

You discover that you are actually taking the examination all the time: you are preparing for the examination by "taking" an examination, not by reading extraneous and/or supererogatory textbooks.

In short, this PASSBOOK®, used directedly, should be an important factor in helping you to pass your test.

Entrance Examinations for Schools of Registered and Practical Nursing

GENERAL

The Entrance Examinations for schools of registered and practical nursing are given throughout the year at established testing centers.

The examinations are designed to aid the schools in selection; there is no passing or failing grade. Results supplement information the schools already have, such as high school grades, etc.

Reports are sent to the schools of nursing within ten days of the date of testing. The reports are sent only to those schools of nursing which have signed the application cards. Reports cannot be sent to the applicants, their parents, their high schools, or any other agency. Only the school of nursing can advise you whether you have been accepted or not; do not write or call the testing organization for this information.

Examinations begin promptly at the scheduled time, so arrive at the testing room about ten minutes before that hour. You may not be allowed to take the examination if you are late.

The test takes approximately 2 hours, including a rest period. During the examination, telephone messages will not be accepted. It is impossible for anyone to wait for you in the testing center while you are taking the test.

APPLICATION PROCEDURE

Obtain an application card from the school of nursing to which you are applying. This card must be signed by the school authorizing you to take the examination.

Print clearly or type all information. Fill in both sides of the application card completely.

1. Use your full name throughout.
2. Address should be the complete address at which you receive your mail.
3. Write your legal signature where required.

Select a testing city and date from the schedule. If your application is not received in time to schedule you for the date you have selected, you will be assigned to the next available date in the same city.

If you have not received an acknowledgment of your application within two weeks, inform the testing organization. The fee for the given examination entitles you to have one report sent to a school of practical or registered nursing.

No application will be processed unless the application card and fee are received at the same time.

The entrance examinations for practical nursing and registered nursing are different and are not interchangeable. Reports of an examination taken for one program will not be sent to the other.

Change of Testing Date

It is possible to change the date and place of testing by sending in a written request with a required fee.

Additional Reports

These may be requested either at the time the original application is made or at any time thereafter.

1. Each request must be accompanied by a required fee.
2. The request for an additional report will not be acknowledged. The report will be sent to the school specified.
3. Indicate whether you have already taken the examination or give the date you plan to take it.

ADMISSION TO THE EXAMINATION

An admission card will be sent to you when the application card and fee are received. Although more than one application card may be received, only one admission card will be issued. The admission card will tell you the exact time and address of the examination. All examinations are scheduled for local time.

The date on which your application card was issued to you is shown on the last line of the card. If you hold your card too long and miss a scheduled testing, an additional fee may be charged.

Examinations can sometimes be arranged in places other than those listed on the schedule. If it is impossible for you to go to a scheduled examination, send your application card, your fee, and a note of explanation to the testing service. Special examinations require an additional fee, but arrangements for them cannot be made until your application card and basic fee are received.

Do not write or call the place of testing. Address all requests for information to the testing service. Enclose a stamped, self-addressed envelope for your reply.

Do not send your fee in cash; use a check or money order. Take several well-sharpened #2 pencils to the testing. No refunds of fees will be made.

Sample Questions

The examinations measure abilities in the following areas. An example of each is shown:

Verbal Ability

Choose the numbered word which means the SAME, or MOST NEARLY the same, as the word given in capitals.

1. IMPEDE

1) approach   2) propel   3) mimic   4) obstruct

Choose the numbered word which means the OPPOSITE, or MOST NEARLY the opposite, of the word given in capitals.

2. CONCUR

1) excuse   2) yield   3) dissent   4) occur

Arithmetic Processes

3. Select the CORRECT answer to the stated problem: .072 =

1) .0072%   2) .072%   3) .72%   4) 7.2%

Quantitative Reasoning

4. If one-sixth of a number plus 3 times the number equals 76, what is the number?

1) 18   2) 22   3) 24   4) 26

Life Sciences

Select the BEST answer from among the four options supplied for each item.

5. The only nutrients which contain nitrogen are

1. fat
2. proteins
3. mineral salts
4. carbohydrates

Physical Sciences

6. Xenon, krypton, radon, and helium are relatively unreactive in chemical reactions because they

    1. contain strong bonds
    2. have low ionization potentials
    3. are gaseous at room temperature
    4. contain filled outer octets of electrons

Reading Comprehension

Read the following passage carefully; then select the BEST answer to the question based on it.

> Thallium sulfate, an inexpensive salt of a metal akin to lead, is one of the most potent poisons that man has developed to combat insects and rodents. Vermin are highly attracted to it; they continue nibbling doughnut-shaped baits containing the poison until they have absorbed a fatal dose. Children, however, are likely to do the same. Cases of this fatal poisoning have been repeated in every state, but they are most common in the South where pesticides are most needed. In 1957, Texas reduced the legal dosage of thallium sulfate in a rat poison mixture from three percent to one percent; in 1960, the federal government did the same, but even the weaker mixture is dangerous and can be deadly. Children who survive accidental poisoning may, months or years later, suffer from uncontrolled and abnormal movements, severe mental illness, or retardation.

7. According to the passage, one result of thallium sulfate poisoning is

    1. paralysis
    2. vomiting
    3. convulsions
    4. difficulty in breaking

KEY (CORRECT ANSWERS)

1.	4	4.	3
2.	3	5.	2
3.	4	6.	4
		7.	3

HOW TO TAKE A TEST

I. YOU MUST PASS AN EXAMINATION

A. WHAT EVERY CANDIDATE SHOULD KNOW

Examination applicants often ask us for help in preparing for the written test. What can I study in advance? What kinds of questions will be asked? How will the test be given? How will the papers be graded?

As an applicant for a civil service examination, you may be wondering about some of these things. Our purpose here is to suggest effective methods of advance study and to describe civil service examinations.

Your chances for success on this examination can be increased if you know how to prepare. Those "pre-examination jitters" can be reduced if you know what to expect. You can even experience an adventure in good citizenship if you know why civil service exams are given.

B. WHY ARE CIVIL SERVICE EXAMINATIONS GIVEN?

Civil service examinations are important to you in two ways. As a citizen, you want public jobs filled by employees who know how to do their work. As a job seeker, you want a fair chance to compete for that job on an equal footing with other candidates. The best-known means of accomplishing this two-fold goal is the competitive examination.

Exams are widely publicized throughout the nation. They may be administered for jobs in federal, state, city, municipal, town or village governments or agencies.

Any citizen may apply, with some limitations, such as the age or residence of applicants. Your experience and education may be reviewed to see whether you meet the requirements for the particular examination. When these requirements exist, they are reasonable and applied consistently to all applicants. Thus, a competitive examination may cause you some uneasiness now, but it is your privilege and safeguard.

C. HOW ARE CIVIL SERVICE EXAMS DEVELOPED?

Examinations are carefully written by trained technicians who are specialists in the field known as "psychological measurement," in consultation with recognized authorities in the field of work that the test will cover. These experts recommend the subject matter areas or skills to be tested; only those knowledges or skills important to your success on the job are included. The most reliable books and source materials available are used as references. Together, the experts and technicians judge the difficulty level of the questions.

Test technicians know how to phrase questions so that the problem is clearly stated. Their ethics do not permit "trick" or "catch" questions. Questions may have been tried out on sample groups, or subjected to statistical analysis, to determine their usefulness.

Written tests are often used in combination with performance tests, ratings of training and experience, and oral interviews. All of these measures combine to form the best-known means of finding the right person for the right job.

II. HOW TO PASS THE WRITTEN TEST

A. NATURE OF THE EXAMINATION

To prepare intelligently for civil service examinations, you should know how they differ from school examinations you have taken. In school you were assigned certain definite pages to read or subjects to cover. The examination questions were quite detailed and usually emphasized memory. Civil service exams, on the other hand, try to discover your present ability to perform the duties of a position, plus your potentiality to learn these duties. In other words, a civil service exam attempts to predict how successful you will be. Questions cover such a broad area that they cannot be as minute and detailed as school exam questions.

In the public service similar kinds of work, or positions, are grouped together in one "class." This process is known as *position-classification*. All the positions in a class are paid according to the salary range for that class. One class title covers all of these positions, and they are all tested by the same examination.

B. FOUR BASIC STEPS

1) Study the announcement

How, then, can you know what subjects to study? Our best answer is: "Learn as much as possible about the class of positions for which you've applied." The exam will test the knowledge, skills and abilities needed to do the work.

Your most valuable source of information about the position you want is the official exam announcement. This announcement lists the training and experience qualifications. Check these standards and apply only if you come reasonably close to meeting them.

The brief description of the position in the examination announcement offers some clues to the subjects which will be tested. Think about the job itself. Review the duties in your mind. Can you perform them, or are there some in which you are rusty? Fill in the blank spots in your preparation.

Many jurisdictions preview the written test in the exam announcement by including a section called "Knowledge and Abilities Required," "Scope of the Examination," or some similar heading. Here you will find out specifically what fields will be tested.

2) Review your own background

Once you learn in general what the position is all about, and what you need to know to do the work, ask yourself which subjects you already know fairly well and which need improvement. You may wonder whether to concentrate on improving your strong areas or on building some background in your fields of weakness. When the announcement has specified "some knowledge" or "considerable knowledge," or has used adjectives like "beginning principles of…" or "advanced … methods," you can get a clue as to the number and difficulty of questions to be asked in any given field. More questions, and hence broader coverage, would be included for those subjects which are more important in the work. Now weigh your strengths and weaknesses against the job requirements and prepare accordingly.

3) Determine the level of the position

Another way to tell how intensively you should prepare is to understand the level of the job for which you are applying. Is it the entering level? In other words, is this the position in which beginners in a field of work are hired? Or is it an intermediate or advanced level? Sometimes this is indicated by such words as "Junior" or "Senior" in the class title. Other jurisdictions use Roman numerals to designate the level – Clerk I, Clerk II, for example. The word "Supervisor" sometimes appears in the title. If the level is not indicated by the title, check the description of duties. Will you be working under very close supervision, or will you have responsibility for independent decisions in this work?

4) Choose appropriate study materials

Now that you know the subjects to be examined and the relative amount of each subject to be covered, you can choose suitable study materials. For beginning level jobs, or even advanced ones, if you have a pronounced weakness in some aspect of your training, read a modern, standard textbook in that field. Be sure it is up to date and has general coverage. Such books are normally available at your library, and the librarian will be glad to help you locate one. For entry-level positions, questions of appropriate difficulty are chosen – neither highly advanced questions, nor those too simple. Such questions require careful thought but not advanced training.

If the position for which you are applying is technical or advanced, you will read more advanced, specialized material. If you are already familiar with the basic principles of your field, elementary textbooks would waste your time. Concentrate on advanced textbooks and technical periodicals. Think through the concepts and review difficult problems in your field.

These are all general sources. You can get more ideas on your own initiative, following these leads. For example, training manuals and publications of the government agency which employs workers in your field can be useful, particularly for technical and professional positions. A letter or visit to the government department involved may result in more specific study suggestions, and certainly will provide you with a more definite idea of the exact nature of the position you are seeking.

III. KINDS OF TESTS

Tests are used for purposes other than measuring knowledge and ability to perform specified duties. For some positions, it is equally important to test ability to make adjustments to new situations or to profit from training. In others, basic mental abilities not dependent on information are essential. Questions which test these things may not appear as pertinent to the duties of the position as those which test for knowledge and information. Yet they are often highly important parts of a fair examination. For very general questions, it is almost impossible to help you direct your study efforts. What we can do is to point out some of the more common of these general abilities needed in public service positions and describe some typical questions.

1) General information

Broad, general information has been found useful for predicting job success in some kinds of work. This is tested in a variety of ways, from vocabulary lists to questions about current events. Basic background in some field of work, such as sociology or economics, may be sampled in a group of questions. Often these are principles which have become familiar to most persons through exposure rather than through formal training. It is difficult to advise you how to study for these questions; being alert to the world around you is our best suggestion.

2) Verbal ability

An example of an ability needed in many positions is verbal or language ability. Verbal ability is, in brief, the ability to use and understand words. Vocabulary and grammar tests are typical measures of this ability. Reading comprehension or paragraph interpretation questions are common in many kinds of civil service tests. You are given a paragraph of written material and asked to find its central meaning.

3) Numerical ability

Number skills can be tested by the familiar arithmetic problem, by checking paired lists of numbers to see which are alike and which are different, or by interpreting charts and graphs. In the latter test, a graph may be printed in the test booklet which you are asked to use as the basis for answering questions.

4) Observation

A popular test for law-enforcement positions is the observation test. A picture is shown to you for several minutes, then taken away. Questions about the picture test your ability to observe both details and larger elements.

5) Following directions

In many positions in the public service, the employee must be able to carry out written instructions dependably and accurately. You may be given a chart with several columns, each column listing a variety of information. The questions require you to carry out directions involving the information given in the chart.

6) Skills and aptitudes

Performance tests effectively measure some manual skills and aptitudes. When the skill is one in which you are trained, such as typing or shorthand, you can practice. These tests are often very much like those given in business school or high school courses. For many of the other skills and aptitudes, however, no short-time preparation can be made. Skills and abilities natural to you or that you have developed throughout your lifetime are being tested.

Many of the general questions just described provide all the data needed to answer the questions and ask you to use your reasoning ability to find the answers. Your best preparation for these tests, as well as for tests of facts and ideas, is to be at your physical and mental best. You, no doubt, have your own methods of getting into an exam-taking mood and keeping "in shape." The next section lists some ideas on this subject.

IV. KINDS OF QUESTIONS

Only rarely is the "essay" question, which you answer in narrative form, used in civil service tests. Civil service tests are usually of the short-answer type. Full instructions for answering these questions will be given to you at the examination. But in case this is your first experience with short-answer questions and separate answer sheets, here is what you need to know:

1) Multiple-choice Questions

Most popular of the short-answer questions is the "multiple choice" or "best answer" question. It can be used, for example, to test for factual knowledge, ability to solve problems or judgment in meeting situations found at work.

A multiple-choice question is normally one of three types—
- It can begin with an incomplete statement followed by several possible endings. You are to find the one ending which *best* completes the statement, although some of the others may not be entirely wrong.
- It can also be a complete statement in the form of a question which is answered by choosing one of the statements listed.

- It can be in the form of a problem – again you select the best answer.

Here is an example of a multiple-choice question with a discussion which should give you some clues as to the method for choosing the right answer:

When an employee has a complaint about his assignment, the action which will *best* help him overcome his difficulty is to
    A. discuss his difficulty with his coworkers
    B. take the problem to the head of the organization
    C. take the problem to the person who gave him the assignment
    D. say nothing to anyone about his complaint

In answering this question, you should study each of the choices to find which is best. Consider choice "A" – Certainly an employee may discuss his complaint with fellow employees, but no change or improvement can result, and the complaint remains unresolved. Choice "B" is a poor choice since the head of the organization probably does not know what assignment you have been given, and taking your problem to him is known as "going over the head" of the supervisor. The supervisor, or person who made the assignment, is the person who can clarify it or correct any injustice. Choice "C" is, therefore, correct. To say nothing, as in choice "D," is unwise. Supervisors have and interest in knowing the problems employees are facing, and the employee is seeking a solution to his problem.

2) True/False Questions

The "true/false" or "right/wrong" form of question is sometimes used. Here a complete statement is given. Your job is to decide whether the statement is right or wrong.

SAMPLE: A roaming cell-phone call to a nearby city costs less than a non-roaming call to a distant city.

This statement is wrong, or false, since roaming calls are more expensive.

This is not a complete list of all possible question forms, although most of the others are variations of these common types. You will always get complete directions for answering questions. Be sure you understand *how* to mark your answers – ask questions until you do.

V. RECORDING YOUR ANSWERS

Computer terminals are used more and more today for many different kinds of exams.
For an examination with very few applicants, you may be told to record your answers in the test booklet itself. Separate answer sheets are much more common. If this separate answer sheet is to be scored by machine – and this is often the case – it is highly important that you mark your answers correctly in order to get credit.
An electronic scoring machine is often used in civil service offices because of the speed with which papers can be scored. Machine-scored answer sheets must be marked with a pencil, which will be given to you. This pencil has a high graphite content which responds to the electronic scoring machine. As a matter of fact, stray dots may register as answers, so do not let your pencil rest on the answer sheet while you are pondering the correct answer. Also, if your pencil lead breaks or is otherwise defective, ask for another.

Since the answer sheet will be dropped in a slot in the scoring machine, be careful not to bend the corners or get the paper crumpled.

The answer sheet normally has five vertical columns of numbers, with 30 numbers to a column. These numbers correspond to the question numbers in your test booklet. After each number, going across the page are four or five pairs of dotted lines. These short dotted lines have small letters or numbers above them. The first two pairs may also have a "T" or "F" above the letters. This indicates that the first two pairs only are to be used if the questions are of the true-false type. If the questions are multiple choice, disregard the "T" and "F" and pay attention only to the small letters or numbers.

Answer your questions in the manner of the sample that follows:

32. The largest city in the United States is
    A. Washington, D.C.
    B. New York City
    C. Chicago
    D. Detroit
    E. San Francisco

1) Choose the answer you think is best. (New York City is the largest, so "B" is correct.)
2) Find the row of dotted lines numbered the same as the question you are answering. (Find row number 32)
3) Find the pair of dotted lines corresponding to the answer. (Find the pair of lines under the mark "B.")
4) Make a solid black mark between the dotted lines.

VI. BEFORE THE TEST

Common sense will help you find procedures to follow to get ready for an examination. Too many of us, however, overlook these sensible measures. Indeed, nervousness and fatigue have been found to be the most serious reasons why applicants fail to do their best on civil service tests. Here is a list of reminders:

- Begin your preparation early – Don't wait until the last minute to go scurrying around for books and materials or to find out what the position is all about.
- Prepare continuously – An hour a night for a week is better than an all-night cram session. This has been definitely established. What is more, a night a week for a month will return better dividends than crowding your study into a shorter period of time.
- Locate the place of the exam – You have been sent a notice telling you when and where to report for the examination. If the location is in a different town or otherwise unfamiliar to you, it would be well to inquire the best route and learn something about the building.
- Relax the night before the test – Allow your mind to rest. Do not study at all that night. Plan some mild recreation or diversion; then go to bed early and get a good night's sleep.
- Get up early enough to make a leisurely trip to the place for the test – This way unforeseen events, traffic snarls, unfamiliar buildings, etc. will not upset you.
- Dress comfortably – A written test is not a fashion show. You will be known by number and not by name, so wear something comfortable.

- Leave excess paraphernalia at home – Shopping bags and odd bundles will get in your way. You need bring only the items mentioned in the official notice you received; usually everything you need is provided. Do not bring reference books to the exam. They will only confuse those last minutes and be taken away from you when in the test room.
- Arrive somewhat ahead of time – If because of transportation schedules you must get there very early, bring a newspaper or magazine to take your mind off yourself while waiting.
- Locate the examination room – When you have found the proper room, you will be directed to the seat or part of the room where you will sit. Sometimes you are given a sheet of instructions to read while you are waiting. Do not fill out any forms until you are told to do so; just read them and be prepared.
- Relax and prepare to listen to the instructions
- If you have any physical problem that may keep you from doing your best, be sure to tell the test administrator. If you are sick or in poor health, you really cannot do your best on the exam. You can come back and take the test some other time.

VII. AT THE TEST

The day of the test is here and you have the test booklet in your hand. The temptation to get going is very strong. Caution! There is more to success than knowing the right answers. You must know how to identify your papers and understand variations in the type of short-answer question used in this particular examination. Follow these suggestions for maximum results from your efforts:

1) Cooperate with the monitor

The test administrator has a duty to create a situation in which you can be as much at ease as possible. He will give instructions, tell you when to begin, check to see that you are marking your answer sheet correctly, and so on. He is not there to guard you, although he will see that your competitors do not take unfair advantage. He wants to help you do your best.

2) Listen to all instructions

Don't jump the gun! Wait until you understand all directions. In most civil service tests you get more time than you need to answer the questions. So don't be in a hurry. Read each word of instructions until you clearly understand the meaning. Study the examples, listen to all announcements and follow directions. Ask questions if you do not understand what to do.

3) Identify your papers

Civil service exams are usually identified by number only. You will be assigned a number; you must not put your name on your test papers. Be sure to copy your number correctly. Since more than one exam may be given, copy your exact examination title.

4) Plan your time

Unless you are told that a test is a "speed" or "rate of work" test, speed itself is usually not important. Time enough to answer all the questions will be provided, but this does not mean that you have all day. An overall time limit has been set. Divide the total time (in minutes) by the number of questions to determine the approximate time you have for each question.

5) Do not linger over difficult questions

If you come across a difficult question, mark it with a paper clip (useful to have along) and come back to it when you have been through the booklet. One caution if you do this – be sure to skip a number on your answer sheet as well. Check often to be sure that you have not lost your place and that you are marking in the row numbered the same as the question you are answering.

6) Read the questions

Be sure you know what the question asks! Many capable people are unsuccessful because they failed to *read* the questions correctly.

7) Answer all questions

Unless you have been instructed that a penalty will be deducted for incorrect answers, it is better to guess than to omit a question.

8) Speed tests

It is often better NOT to guess on speed tests. It has been found that on timed tests people are tempted to spend the last few seconds before time is called in marking answers at random – without even reading them – in the hope of picking up a few extra points. To discourage this practice, the instructions may warn you that your score will be "corrected" for guessing. That is, a penalty will be applied. The incorrect answers will be deducted from the correct ones, or some other penalty formula will be used.

9) Review your answers

If you finish before time is called, go back to the questions you guessed or omitted to give them further thought. Review other answers if you have time.

10) Return your test materials

If you are ready to leave before others have finished or time is called, take ALL your materials to the monitor and leave quietly. Never take any test material with you. The monitor can discover whose papers are not complete, and taking a test booklet may be grounds for disqualification.

VIII. EXAMINATION TECHNIQUES

1) Read the general instructions carefully. These are usually printed on the first page of the exam booklet. As a rule, these instructions refer to the timing of the examination; the fact that you should not start work until the signal and must stop work at a signal, etc. If there are any *special* instructions, such as a choice of questions to be answered, make sure that you note this instruction carefully.

2) When you are ready to start work on the examination, that is as soon as the signal has been given, read the instructions to each question booklet, underline any key words or phrases, such as *least, best, outline, describe* and the like. In this way you will tend to answer as requested rather than discover on reviewing your paper that you *listed without describing*, that you selected the *worst* choice rather than the *best* choice, etc.

3) If the examination is of the objective or multiple-choice type – that is, each question will also give a series of possible answers: A, B, C or D, and you are called upon to select the best answer and write the letter next to that answer on your answer paper – it is advisable to start answering each question in turn. There may be anywhere from 50 to 100 such questions in the three or four hours allotted and you can see how much time would be taken if you read through all the questions before beginning to answer any. Furthermore, if you come across a question or group of questions which you know would be difficult to answer, it would undoubtedly affect your handling of all the other questions.

4) If the examination is of the essay type and contains but a few questions, it is a moot point as to whether you should read all the questions before starting to answer any one. Of course, if you are given a choice – say five out of seven and the like – then it is essential to read all the questions so you can eliminate the two that are most difficult. If, however, you are asked to answer all the questions, there may be danger in trying to answer the easiest one first because you may find that you will spend too much time on it. The best technique is to answer the first question, then proceed to the second, etc.

5) Time your answers. Before the exam begins, write down the time it started, then add the time allowed for the examination and write down the time it must be completed, then divide the time available somewhat as follows:
    - If 3-1/2 hours are allowed, that would be 210 minutes. If you have 80 objective-type questions, that would be an average of 2-1/2 minutes per question. Allow yourself no more than 2 minutes per question, or a total of 160 minutes, which will permit about 50 minutes to review.
    - If for the time allotment of 210 minutes there are 7 essay questions to answer, that would average about 30 minutes a question. Give yourself only 25 minutes per question so that you have about 35 minutes to review.

6) The most important instruction is to *read each question* and make sure you know what is wanted. The second most important instruction is to *time yourself properly* so that you answer every question. The third most important instruction is to *answer every question*. Guess if you have to but include something for each question. Remember that you will receive no credit for a blank and will probably receive some credit if you write something in answer to an essay question. If you guess a letter – say "B" for a multiple-choice question – you may have guessed right. If you leave a blank as an answer to a multiple-choice question, the examiners may respect your feelings but it will not add a point to your score. Some exams may penalize you for wrong answers, so in such cases *only*, you may not want to guess unless you have some basis for your answer.

7) Suggestions
    a. Objective-type questions
        1. Examine the question booklet for proper sequence of pages and questions
        2. Read all instructions carefully
        3. Skip any question which seems too difficult; return to it after all other questions have been answered
        4. Apportion your time properly; do not spend too much time on any single question or group of questions

5. Note and underline key words – *all, most, fewest, least, best, worst, same, opposite,* etc.
6. Pay particular attention to negatives
7. Note unusual option, e.g., unduly long, short, complex, different or similar in content to the body of the question
8. Observe the use of "hedging" words – *probably, may, most likely,* etc.
9. Make sure that your answer is put next to the same number as the question
10. Do not second-guess unless you have good reason to believe the second answer is definitely more correct
11. Cross out original answer if you decide another answer is more accurate; do not erase until you are ready to hand your paper in
12. Answer all questions; guess unless instructed otherwise
13. Leave time for review

b. Essay questions
   1. Read each question carefully
   2. Determine exactly what is wanted. Underline key words or phrases.
   3. Decide on outline or paragraph answer
   4. Include many different points and elements unless asked to develop any one or two points or elements
   5. Show impartiality by giving pros and cons unless directed to select one side only
   6. Make and write down any assumptions you find necessary to answer the questions
   7. Watch your English, grammar, punctuation and choice of words
   8. Time your answers; don't crowd material

8) Answering the essay question

Most essay questions can be answered by framing the specific response around several key words or ideas. Here are a few such key words or ideas:

M's: manpower, materials, methods, money, management
P's: purpose, program, policy, plan, procedure, practice, problems, pitfalls, personnel, public relations
   a. Six basic steps in handling problems:
      1. Preliminary plan and background development
      2. Collect information, data and facts
      3. Analyze and interpret information, data and facts
      4. Analyze and develop solutions as well as make recommendations
      5. Prepare report and sell recommendations
      6. Install recommendations and follow up effectiveness

   b. Pitfalls to avoid
      1. *Taking things for granted* – A statement of the situation does not necessarily imply that each of the elements is necessarily true; for example, a complaint may be invalid and biased so that all that can be taken for granted is that a complaint has been registered

2. *Considering only one side of a situation* – Wherever possible, indicate several alternatives and then point out the reasons you selected the best one
3. *Failing to indicate follow up* – Whenever your answer indicates action on your part, make certain that you will take proper follow-up action to see how successful your recommendations, procedures or actions turn out to be
4. *Taking too long in answering any single question* – Remember to time your answers properly

IX. AFTER THE TEST

Scoring procedures differ in detail among civil service jurisdictions although the general principles are the same. Whether the papers are hand-scored or graded by machine we have described, they are nearly always graded by number. That is, the person who marks the paper knows only the number – never the name – of the applicant. Not until all the papers have been graded will they be matched with names. If other tests, such as training and experience or oral interview ratings have been given, scores will be combined. Different parts of the examination usually have different weights. For example, the written test might count 60 percent of the final grade, and a rating of training and experience 40 percent. In many jurisdictions, veterans will have a certain number of points added to their grades.

After the final grade has been determined, the names are placed in grade order and an eligible list is established. There are various methods for resolving ties between those who get the same final grade – probably the most common is to place first the name of the person whose application was received first. Job offers are made from the eligible list in the order the names appear on it. You will be notified of your grade and your rank as soon as all these computations have been made. This will be done as rapidly as possible.

People who are found to meet the requirements in the announcement are called "eligibles." Their names are put on a list of eligible candidates. An eligible's chances of getting a job depend on how high he stands on this list and how fast agencies are filling jobs from the list.

When a job is to be filled from a list of eligibles, the agency asks for the names of people on the list of eligibles for that job. When the civil service commission receives this request, it sends to the agency the names of the three people highest on this list. Or, if the job to be filled has specialized requirements, the office sends the agency the names of the top three persons who meet these requirements from the general list.

The appointing officer makes a choice from among the three people whose names were sent to him. If the selected person accepts the appointment, the names of the others are put back on the list to be considered for future openings.

That is the rule in hiring from all kinds of eligible lists, whether they are for typist, carpenter, chemist, or something else. For every vacancy, the appointing officer has his choice of any one of the top three eligibles on the list. This explains why the person whose name is on top of the list sometimes does not get an appointment when some of the persons lower on the list do. If the appointing officer chooses the second or third eligible, the No. 1 eligible does not get a job at once, but stays on the list until he is appointed or the list is terminated.

X. HOW TO PASS THE INTERVIEW TEST

The examination for which you applied requires an oral interview test. You have already taken the written test and you are now being called for the interview test – the final part of the formal examination.

You may think that it is not possible to prepare for an interview test and that there are no procedures to follow during an interview. Our purpose is to point out some things you can do in advance that will help you and some good rules to follow and pitfalls to avoid while you are being interviewed.

What is an interview supposed to test?

The written examination is designed to test the technical knowledge and competence of the candidate; the oral is designed to evaluate intangible qualities, not readily measured otherwise, and to establish a list showing the relative fitness of each candidate – as measured against his competitors – for the position sought. Scoring is not on the basis of "right" and "wrong," but on a sliding scale of values ranging from "not passable" to "outstanding." As a matter of fact, it is possible to achieve a relatively low score without a single "incorrect" answer because of evident weakness in the qualities being measured.

Occasionally, an examination may consist entirely of an oral test – either an individual or a group oral. In such cases, information is sought concerning the technical knowledges and abilities of the candidate, since there has been no written examination for this purpose. More commonly, however, an oral test is used to supplement a written examination.

Who conducts interviews?

The composition of oral boards varies among different jurisdictions. In nearly all, a representative of the personnel department serves as chairman. One of the members of the board may be a representative of the department in which the candidate would work. In some cases, "outside experts" are used, and, frequently, a businessman or some other representative of the general public is asked to serve. Labor and management or other special groups may be represented. The aim is to secure the services of experts in the appropriate field.

However the board is composed, it is a good idea (and not at all improper or unethical) to ascertain in advance of the interview who the members are and what groups they represent. When you are introduced to them, you will have some idea of their backgrounds and interests, and at least you will not stutter and stammer over their names.

What should be done before the interview?

While knowledge about the board members is useful and takes some of the surprise element out of the interview, there is other preparation which is more substantive. It *is* possible to prepare for an oral interview – in several ways:

1) Keep a copy of your application and review it carefully before the interview

This may be the only document before the oral board, and the starting point of the interview. Know what education and experience you have listed there, and the sequence and dates of all of it. Sometimes the board will ask you to review the highlights of your experience for them; you should not have to hem and haw doing it.

2) Study the class specification and the examination announcement

Usually, the oral board has one or both of these to guide them. The qualities, characteristics or knowledges required by the position sought are stated in these documents. They offer valuable clues as to the nature of the oral interview. For example, if the job involves supervisory responsibilities, the announcement will usually indicate that knowledge of modern supervisory methods and the qualifications of the candidate as a supervisor will be tested. If so, you can expect such questions, frequently in the form of a hypothetical situation which you are expected to solve. NEVER go into an oral without knowledge of the duties and responsibilities of the job you seek.

3) Think through each qualification required

Try to visualize the kind of questions you would ask if you were a board member. How well could you answer them? Try especially to appraise your own knowledge and background in each area, *measured against the job sought*, and identify any areas in which you are weak. Be critical and realistic – do not flatter yourself.

4) Do some general reading in areas in which you feel you may be weak

For example, if the job involves supervision and your past experience has NOT, some general reading in supervisory methods and practices, particularly in the field of human relations, might be useful. Do NOT study agency procedures or detailed manuals. The oral board will be testing your understanding and capacity, not your memory.

5) Get a good night's sleep and watch your general health and mental attitude

You will want a clear head at the interview. Take care of a cold or any other minor ailment, and of course, no hangovers.

What should be done on the day of the interview?

Now comes the day of the interview itself. Give yourself plenty of time to get there. Plan to arrive somewhat ahead of the scheduled time, particularly if your appointment is in the fore part of the day. If a previous candidate fails to appear, the board might be ready for you a bit early. By early afternoon an oral board is almost invariably behind schedule if there are many candidates, and you may have to wait. Take along a book or magazine to read, or your application to review, but leave any extraneous material in the waiting room when you go in for your interview. In any event, relax and compose yourself.

The matter of dress is important. The board is forming impressions about you – from your experience, your manners, your attitude, and your appearance. Give your personal appearance careful attention. Dress your best, but not your flashiest. Choose conservative, appropriate clothing, and be sure it is immaculate. This is a business interview, and your appearance should indicate that you regard it as such. Besides, being well groomed and properly dressed will help boost your confidence.

Sooner or later, someone will call your name and escort you into the interview room. *This is it.* From here on you are on your own. It is too late for any more preparation. But remember, you asked for this opportunity to prove your fitness, and you are here because your request was granted.

What happens when you go in?

The usual sequence of events will be as follows: The clerk (who is often the board stenographer) will introduce you to the chairman of the oral board, who will introduce you to the other members of the board. Acknowledge the introductions before you sit down. Do not be surprised if you find a microphone facing you or a stenotypist sitting by. Oral interviews are usually recorded in the event of an appeal or other review.

Usually the chairman of the board will open the interview by reviewing the highlights of your education and work experience from your application – primarily for the benefit of the other members of the board, as well as to get the material into the record. Do not interrupt or comment unless there is an error or significant misinterpretation; if that is the case, do not hesitate. But do not quibble about insignificant matters. Also, he will usually ask you some question about your education, experience or your present job – partly to get you to start talking and to establish the interviewing "rapport." He may start the actual questioning, or turn it over to one of the other members. Frequently, each member undertakes the questioning on a particular area, one in which he is perhaps most competent, so you can expect each member to participate in the examination. Because time is limited, you may also expect some rather abrupt switches in the direction the questioning takes, so do not be upset by it. Normally, a board member will not pursue a single line of questioning unless he discovers a particular strength or weakness.

After each member has participated, the chairman will usually ask whether any member has any further questions, then will ask you if you have anything you wish to add. Unless you are expecting this question, it may floor you. Worse, it may start you off on an extended, extemporaneous speech. The board is not usually seeking more information. The question is principally to offer you a last opportunity to present further qualifications or to indicate that you have nothing to add. So, if you feel that a significant qualification or characteristic has been overlooked, it is proper to point it out in a sentence or so. Do not compliment the board on the thoroughness of their examination – they have been sketchy, and you know it. If you wish, merely say, "No thank you, I have nothing further to add." This is a point where you can "talk yourself out" of a good impression or fail to present an important bit of information. Remember, *you close the interview yourself.*

The chairman will then say, "That is all, Mr. _____, thank you." Do not be startled; the interview is over, and quicker than you think. Thank him, gather your belongings and take your leave. Save your sigh of relief for the other side of the door.

How to put your best foot forward

Throughout this entire process, you may feel that the board individually and collectively is trying to pierce your defenses, seek out your hidden weaknesses and embarrass and confuse you. Actually, this is not true. They are obliged to make an appraisal of your qualifications for the job you are seeking, and they want to see you in your best light. Remember, they must interview all candidates and a non-cooperative candidate may become a failure in spite of their best efforts to bring out his qualifications. Here are 15 suggestions that will help you:

1) Be natural – Keep your attitude confident, not cocky

If you are not confident that you can do the job, do not expect the board to be. Do not apologize for your weaknesses, try to bring out your strong points. The board is interested in a positive, not negative, presentation. Cockiness will antagonize any board member and make him wonder if you are covering up a weakness by a false show of strength.

2) Get comfortable, but don't lounge or sprawl

Sit erectly but not stiffly. A careless posture may lead the board to conclude that you are careless in other things, or at least that you are not impressed by the importance of the occasion. Either conclusion is natural, even if incorrect. Do not fuss with your clothing, a pencil or an ashtray. Your hands may occasionally be useful to emphasize a point; do not let them become a point of distraction.

3) Do not wisecrack or make small talk

This is a serious situation, and your attitude should show that you consider it as such. Further, the time of the board is limited – they do not want to waste it, and neither should you.

4) Do not exaggerate your experience or abilities
   In the first place, from information in the application or other interviews and sources, the board may know more about you than you think. Secondly, you probably will not get away with it. An experienced board is rather adept at spotting such a situation, so do not take the chance.

5) If you know a board member, do not make a point of it, yet do not hide it
   Certainly you are not fooling him, and probably not the other members of the board. Do not try to take advantage of your acquaintanceship – it will probably do you little good.

6) Do not dominate the interview
   Let the board do that. They will give you the clues – do not assume that you have to do all the talking. Realize that the board has a number of questions to ask you, and do not try to take up all the interview time by showing off your extensive knowledge of the answer to the first one.

7) Be attentive
   You only have 20 minutes or so, and you should keep your attention at its sharpest throughout. When a member is addressing a problem or question to you, give him your undivided attention. Address your reply principally to him, but do not exclude the other board members.

8) Do not interrupt
   A board member may be stating a problem for you to analyze. He will ask you a question when the time comes. Let him state the problem, and wait for the question.

9) Make sure you understand the question
   Do not try to answer until you are sure what the question is. If it is not clear, restate it in your own words or ask the board member to clarify it for you. However, do not haggle about minor elements.

10) Reply promptly but not hastily
   A common entry on oral board rating sheets is "candidate responded readily," or "candidate hesitated in replies." Respond as promptly and quickly as you can, but do not jump to a hasty, ill-considered answer.

11) Do not be peremptory in your answers
   A brief answer is proper – but do not fire your answer back. That is a losing game from your point of view. The board member can probably ask questions much faster than you can answer them.

12) Do not try to create the answer you think the board member wants
   He is interested in what kind of mind you have and how it works – not in playing games. Furthermore, he can usually spot this practice and will actually grade you down on it.

13) Do not switch sides in your reply merely to agree with a board member
   Frequently, a member will take a contrary position merely to draw you out and to see if you are willing and able to defend your point of view. Do not start a debate, yet do not surrender a good position. If a position is worth taking, it is worth defending.

14) Do not be afraid to admit an error in judgment if you are shown to be wrong

The board knows that you are forced to reply without any opportunity for careful consideration. Your answer may be demonstrably wrong. If so, admit it and get on with the interview.

15) Do not dwell at length on your present job

The opening question may relate to your present assignment. Answer the question but do not go into an extended discussion. You are being examined for a *new* job, not your present one. As a matter of fact, try to phrase ALL your answers in terms of the job for which you are being examined.

Basis of Rating

Probably you will forget most of these "do's" and "don'ts" when you walk into the oral interview room. Even remembering them all will not ensure you a passing grade. Perhaps you did not have the qualifications in the first place. But remembering them will help you to put your best foot forward, without treading on the toes of the board members.

Rumor and popular opinion to the contrary notwithstanding, an oral board wants you to make the best appearance possible. They know you are under pressure – but they also want to see how you respond to it as a guide to what your reaction would be under the pressures of the job you seek. They will be influenced by the degree of poise you display, the personal traits you show and the manner in which you respond.

ABOUT THIS BOOK

This book contains tests divided into Examination Sections. Go through each test, answering every question in the margin. We have also attached a sample answer sheet at the back of the book that can be removed and used. At the end of each test look at the answer key and check your answers. On the ones you got wrong, look at the right answer choice and learn. Do not fill in the answers first. Do not memorize the questions and answers, but understand the answer and principles involved. On your test, the questions will likely be different from the samples. Questions are changed and new ones added. If you understand these past questions you should have success with any changes that arise. Tests may consist of several types of questions. We have additional books on each subject should more study be advisable or necessary for you. Finally, the more you study, the better prepared you will be. This book is intended to be the last thing you study before you walk into the examination room. Prior study of relevant texts is also recommended. NLC publishes some of these in our Fundamental Series. Knowledge and good sense are important factors in passing your exam. Good luck also helps. So now study this Passbook, absorb the material contained within and take that knowledge into the examination. Then do your best to pass that exam.

EXAMINATION SECTION

EXAMINATION SECTION
TEST 1

DIRECTIONS: Each question or incomplete statement is followed by several suggested answers or completions. Select the one that BEST answers the question or completes the statement. *PRINT THE LETTER OF THE CORRECT ANSWER IN THE SPACE AT THE RIGHT.*

Questions 1-10.

DIRECTIONS: In answering Questions 1 through 10, select the alternative that means the *same as* or the *opposite* of the word in italics.

1. *acquire*
   - A. judge
   - B. identify
   - C. surrender
   - D. educate
   - E. happen

2. *begrudge*
   - A. envy
   - B. hate
   - C. annoy
   - D. obstruct
   - E. punish

3. *obsolete*
   - A. fatal
   - B. modern
   - C. distracting
   - D. untouched
   - E. broken

4. *inflexible*
   - A. weak
   - B. righteous
   - C. harmless
   - D. unyielding
   - E. secret

5. *nominal*
   - A. just
   - B. slight
   - C. cheerful
   - D. familiar
   - E. ceaseless

6. *debt*
   - A. insane
   - B. artificial
   - C. skillful
   - D. determined
   - E. humble

7. *censure*
   - A. focus
   - B. exclude
   - C. baffle
   - D. portray
   - E. praise

8. *nebulous*
   - A. imaginary
   - B. spiritual
   - C. distinct
   - D. starry-eyed
   - E. unanswerable

9. *impart*
   - A. hasten
   - B. adjust
   - C. gamble
   - D. address
   - E. communicate

10. *terminate*
    A. gain
    B. graduate
    C. harvest
    D. start
    E. paralyze

Questions 11-20.

DIRECTIONS: In answering Questions 11 through 20, select the word which, if inserted in the blank space, agrees MOST closely with the thought of the sentence.

11. Every good story is carefully contrived; the elements of the story are _____ to fi with one another in order to make an effect on the reader.
    A. read
    B. learned
    C. emphasized
    D. reduced
    E. planned

12. Their work was commemorative in character and consisted largely of _____ erected upon the occasion of victories.
    A. towers
    B. tombs
    C. monuments
    D. castles
    E. fortresses

13. Before criticizing the work of an artist, one needs to _____ the artist's purpose.
    A. understand
    B. reveal
    C. defend
    D. correct
    E. change

14. Because in the administration it hath respect not to the group but to the _____, our form of government is called a democracy.
    A. courts
    B. people
    C. majority
    D. individual
    E. law

15. Deductive reasoning is that form of reasoning in which the conclusion must necessarily follow if we accept the premise as true. In deduction, it is _____ for the premise to be true and the conclusion false.
    A. impossible
    B. inevitable
    C. reasonable
    D. surprising
    E. unlikely

16. Mathematics is the product of thought operating by means of _____ for the purpose of expressing general laws.
    A. reasoning
    B. symbols
    C. words
    D. examples
    E. science

17. No other man loss so much, so _____, so absolutely, as the beaten candidate for high public office.
    A. bewilderingly
    B. predictably
    C. disgracefully
    D. publicly
    E. cheerfully

18. Many television watchers enjoy stories which contain violence. Consequently, those television producers who are dominated by rating systems aim to _____ the popular taste.
    A. raise   B. control   C. gratify
    D. ignore   e. lower

    18.____

19. The latent period for the contractile response to direct stimulation of the muscle has quite another and shorter value, encompassing only a utilization period. Hence, it is that the term *latent period* must be _____ carefully each time that it is used.
    A. checked   B. timed   C. introduced
    D. defined   E. selected

    19.____

20. A man who cannot win honor in his own _____ will have a very small chance of winning it from posterity.
    A. right   B. field   C. country
    D. way   E. age

    20.____

Questions 21-35.

DIRECTIONS: In answering Questions 21 through 35, select the word that BEST completes the analogy.

21. Albino is to color as traitor is to
    A. patriotism   B. treachery   C. socialism
    D. integration E. liberalism

    21.____

22. Senile is to infantile as supper is to
    A. snack   B. breakfast   C. dinner
    D. daytime   E. evening

    22.____

23. Snow shovel is to sidewalk as eraser is to
    A. writing   B. pencil   C. paper
    D. desk   E. mistake

    23.____

24. Lawyer is to court as soldier is to
    A. battle   B. victory   C. training
    D. rifle   E. discipline

    24.____

25. Faucet is to water as mosquito is to
    A. swamp   B. butterfly   C. cistern
    D. pond   E. malaria

    25.____

26. Astronomy is to geology as steeplejack is to
    A. mailman   B. surgeon   C. pilot
    D. miner   E. skindiver

    26.____

27. Chimney is to smoke as guide is to
    A. snare   B. compass   C. hunter
    D. firewood   E. wild game

28. Prodigy is to ability as ocean is to
    A. water   B. waves   C. ships
    D. icebergs   E. current

29. War is to devastation as microbe is to
    A. peace   B. flea   C. dog
    D. germ   E. pestilence

30. Blueberry is to pea a sky is to
    A. storm   B. world   C. star
    D. grass   E. purity

31. Pour is to spill as lie is to
    A. deception   B. misstatement   C. falsehood
    D. perjury   E. fraud

32. Disparage is to despise as praise is to
    A. dislike   B. adore   C. acclaim
    D. advocate   E. compliment

33. Wall is to mortar as nation is to
    A. family   B. people   C. patriotism
    D. geography   E. boundaries

34. Servant is to butter as pain is to
    A. cramp   B. hurt   C. illness
    D. itch   E. anesthesia

35. Fan is to air as newspaper is to
    A. literature   B. reporter   C. information
    D. subscription E. reader

36. A set of papers is arranged and numbered from 1 to 49.
    If the paper numbered 3 is drawn first and every ninth paper thereafter, what will be the number of the last paper drawn?
    A. 45   B. 46   C. 47   D. 48   E. 49

37. Which quantity can be measured *exactly* from a tank of water by using only a 10-pint can and an 8-pint can? _____ pint(s)
    A. 1   B. 6   C. 3   D. 7   E. 5

38. If city R has more fires than city S, and city T has more fires than cities P and S combined, then the number of fires in city
    A. P must be less than in city T
    B. T must be less than in city R
    C. T must be greater than in city R
    D. R must be greater than in city P
    E. S must be greater than in city T

39. The average of three numbers is 25.
    If one of the numbers is increased by 4, the average will remain unchanged if each of the other two numbers is reduced by
    A. 1   B. 2   C. 2/3   D. 4   E. 1 1/3

40.
```
                    1
                 1     1
              1    2    1
           1    3    3    1
        1    4    6    4    1
     1    5   10    X    5    1
```
    Above are the first six rows of a triangular array constructed according to a fixed law.
    What number does the letter X represent?
    A. 8   B. 10   C. 15   D. 20   E. 5

41. If all A are C and no C are B, it necessarily follows that
    A. all B are C   B. all B are A   C. no A are B
    D. no C are A   E. some B are A

42. What number is missing in the series 7, ____, 63, 189?
    A. 9   B. 11   C. 19   D. 21   E. 24

43. A clock that gains one minute each hour is synchronized at noon with a clock that loses two minutes an hour.
    How many minutes apart will the minute hands of the two clocks be at midnight?
    A. 0   B. 12   C. 14   D. 24   E. 30

44. The pages of a typewritten report are numbered by hand from 1 to 100.
    How many times will it be necessary to write the numeral 5?
    A. 10   B. 11   C. 12   D. 19   E. 20

45. The number 6 is called a *perfect* number because it is the sum of all its integral divisors except itself.
    Another *perfect* number is
    A. 12   B. 16   C. 24   D. 28   E. 36

KEY (CORRECT ANSWERS)

1. C	11. E	21. A	31. B	41. C
2. A	12. C	22. B	32. B	42. D
3. B	13. A	23. C	33. C	43. D
4. D	14. D	24. A	34. A	44. E
5. B	15. A	25. E	35. C	45. D
6. C	16. B	26. D	36. D	
7. E	17. D	27. C	37. B	
8. C	18. C	28. A	38. A	
9. E	19. D	29. E	39. B	
10. D	20. E	30. D	40. B	

EXAMINATION SECTION

TEST 1

ENGLISH USAGE

DIRECTIONS: This section is based on passages which contain expressions that are inappropriate in standard written English. You are to decide how these expressions can be made appropriate and effective.

The passages are presented in a spread-out format in which various words, phrases, and punctuation have been underlined and numbered. In the right-hand column, opposite each underlined portion, you will find a set of responses numbered to correspond to that of the underlined portion. Each set of responses contains a NO CHANGE option and three alternatives to the underlined version.

Since your judgment about the appropriateness and effectiveness of a response will depend on your perceptions of the passage as a whole, the author's purpose and the type of audience, first read through the entire passage quickly. Then, reread the passage slowly and carefully. As you come to each underlined portion during your second reading, look at the alternatives in the right-hand column and decide which of the four words or phrasings is BEST for the given context. Since your response will often depend on your reading several of the sentences surrounding the underlined portion, make sure you have read ahead far enough to make the best choice.

If you think that the original version (the one in the passage) is best, indicate A in the corresponding space at the right. If you think that an alternative version is best, indicate the letter corresponding to the alternative that you have chosen as best.

In every case, consider ONLY the underlined words, phrases, and punctuation marks; you can assume that the rest of the passage is correct as written.

Thor Heyerdahl became famous for a unique sailing expedition, which he later described in KON-TIKI. Having developed a theory that the original Polynesians had sailed or drifted to the South Sea Islands from South America, <u>it then had to be tested</u>. After careful study, he built a raft
₁

1. A. NO CHANGE
   B. he set out to test it
   C. it was decided that it must be tested
   D. the theory was then to be tested

1.____

that was as authentic as possible. Using only primitive equipment, he and five other men sailed into the South Seas from <u>Peru, which he judged to be in the same</u> general
₂
area as the land of

2. A. NO CHANGE
   B. Peru, being judged as
   C. Peru, which had been
   D. Peru judged as being

2.____

the original Polynesians. As a result, his group and him will long be remembered not only as thorough scientists but also as courageous men.

    Heyerdahl's courage was first tested in Ecuador. His search for trees that was large enough for the expeditionary raft sent him to Quito, a city high in the Andes. There, he and his companions were warned about headhunters and bandits on the trail. Feeling undaunted, they hired a driver and jeep from the U.S. Embassy, going on with their dangerous task

After the raft was done, Heyerdahl made final preparations for the expedition. Even before his crew came aboard, the courage which Heyerdahl possessed was tested again. As the raft was being towed out of the harbor, it drifted under the stern of a tug. Heyerdahl had to struggle to save it.

Dangers at sea were present, but Heyerdahl and his men did not show fear. Instead they developed games that were actually tests of courage. Although man-eating fish were nearby, the men swam to relieve

3. A. NO CHANGE
   B. him and his group
   C. his group and himself
   D. he and his group

4. A. NO CHANGE
   B. which would be of sufficient size
   C. of adequate size
   D. of certainly sufficient size

5. A. NO CHANGE
   B. trail. Undaunted, they
   C. trail, but they were undaunted, and
   D. trail; undaunted they

6. A. NO CHANAGE
   B. Embassy; and went on with
   C. Embassy and proceeded with
   D. Embassy, and kept on

7. A. NO CHANGE
   B. When the raft was ready
   C. The raft was speedily completed and
   D. The raft having been

8. A. NO CHANGE
   B. Heyerdahls' manly courage
   C. Heyerdahl's courage
   D. the courage of this man

9. A. NO CHANGE
   B. (Do not begin new paragraph) At sea, dangers
   C. (Begin new paragraph) Dangers, at sea
   D. (Begin new paragraph) At sea, dangers

their tension, maintaining that the fish were
                10
not dangerous unless a man had already
been cut or scratched. One game consisted
of luring sharks within reach,

catching them, and then they would yank it
                         11
onto the raft.

Being on the raft, the sharks thrashed about
      12
and snapped viciously at the men. Another
game was even more dangerous: two men
would paddle away on a rubber dinghy until

they could catch only an occasional glimpse
                   13
of the raft, then they would have to paddle
violently to return.

The final portion of the voyage was the most
thrilling. As the raft neared Raoia, it was
carried rapidly toward the reef, where the
waves beat it very bad. Almost miraculously
                 14
the

men survived, only to find themselves on a
                    15
deserted island. At last their struggle with
the sea had ended. They radioed Rarotonga
and set up camp to await rescue,

Thor Heyerdahl's expedition on the Kon-Tiki
did not necessarily prove his migration theory,
but it did prove that hardy pioneers with
courage, determination, and luck could make
the same trip, even with very primitive
   16
equipment.

10. A. NO CHANGE
    B. tension. Maintaining
    C. tension. He maintained
    D. tension, because it was maintained

10.____

11. A. NO CHANGE
    B. then to yank it
    C. and then to yank them up
    D. and yanking them

11.____

12. A. NO CHANGE
    B. At that point,
    C. Once there,
    D. A that time,

12.____

13. A. NO CHANGE
    B. (Place after *until*)
    C. (Place after *they*)
    D. OMIT

13.____

14. A. NO CHANGE
    B. mercilessly
    C. very violent
    D. without any mercy

14.____

15. A. NO CHANGE
    B. and only found themselves
    C. only to find themselves
    D. but only found themselves to be

15.____

16. A. NO CHANGE
    B. could now do the same trip
    C. could do the same
    D. could have accomplished this the same,

KEY (CORRECT ANSWERS)

1. B
2. A
3. D
4. C
5. B
6. C
7. B
8. C
9. D
10. A
11. D
12. C
13. A
14. B
15. C
16. A

TEST 2

MATHEMATICS USAGE

DIRECTIONS: Each question or incomplete statement is followed by several suggested answers or completions. Select the one that BEST answers the question or completes the statement. *PRINT THE LETTER OF THE CORRECT ANSWER IN THE SPACE AT THE RIGHT.*

1. Two wells pump oil continuously. One produces 4,000 barrels of oil per day, which is 33 1/3% more than other well produces.
   How many barrels of oil are produced daily by the two wells?
   A. 5333 1/3   B. 6666 2/3   C. 7000
   D. 8333 1/3   E. 9000

   1.____

2. If a car travels a miles in b minutes, how many minutes will it take to travel c miles?
   A. c/a   B. c/b   C. c/ab   D. ab/c   E. cb/a

   2.____

3. In the figure at the right, what is the sum of the angles labeled x and y?
   A. 90°
   B. 100°
   C. 130°
   D. 140°
   E. None of the above

   3.____

4. A man purchased 100 shares of stock at $5 a share.
   If each share rose 10 cents the first month, decreased 8 cents the second month, and gained 3 cents the third month, what was the value of the man's investment at the end of the third month?
   A. $505   B. $520   C. $525
   D. $1,545   E. None of the above

   4.____

5. $$\Delta \times \theta = \theta$$
   $$\theta \times \Delta = \theta$$
   $$\Delta \times \Delta = \Delta$$
   The above multiplication scheme uses symbols other than the usual numerals. A corresponds to which base-10 numeral?
   A. 0   B. 1   C. 2   D. 5   E. 10

   5.____

6. What is the length, in inches, of a 144 arc in a circle whose circumference is 60 inches?
   A. 24   B. 12/π   C. 12π   D. 36   E. 36/π

   6.____

7. What does x equal in the equation $\frac{1}{x} = \frac{1}{5} \cdot \frac{1}{x}$?

   7.____

8. In the universe of all people, let circle M represent all Mary's friends, circle B all Bill's friends, and circle P all Pete's friends.
What is represented by the shaded portion of the figure?
All the people who are
   A. friends of Mary, Bill, and Pete
   B. friends of Mary and Pete
   C. friends of Mary and Pete, but not of Bill
   D. friends of Pete, but not of Bill
   E. not friends of Bill

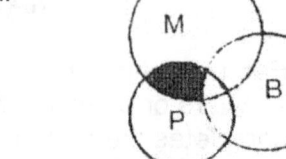

9. A ship sailing due north past an island travels a course that is 12 miles from the island at its closest point.
If a gun on shore has a firing range of 13 miles, for how many miles will the ship remain within range of the gun?
   A. 1
   B. 5
   C. 9
   D. 10
   E. None of the above

10. What is the area of the unshaded sector of circle O shown at the right?
   A. $\dfrac{\pi r}{8}$
   B. $\dfrac{\pi r^2}{2}$
   C. $\dfrac{\pi r^2}{4}$
   D. $\dfrac{\pi r^2}{8}$
   E. $\dfrac{\pi r^2}{45}$

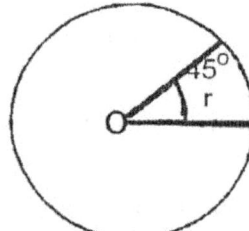

11. What set of values for x and y(x,y) satisfy the following equations: $3y = x + 4$, $6x + 2y = 16$?
   A. (-2,2)
   B. (2,-2)
   C. (-2,2)
   D. (2,2)
   E. None of the above

12. What is the value of the following expression $\dfrac{A^{4}p+3 \cdot A^{3}p+4}{A^{2}p+2}$?

   A. A^{9P+9}
   B. A^{6P+6}
   C. A^{3P+3}
   D. A^{-3P-3}
   E. A^{5P+5}

KEY (CORRECT ANSWERS)

1.	C	7.	D
2.	E	8.	C
3.	A	9.	D
4.	A	10.	D
5.	B	11	D
6.	A	12.	E

TEST 3

SOCIAL STUDIES READING

DIRECTIONS: This test measures your ability to comprehend, analyze, and evaluate reading, materials in such social studies fields as history, political science, economics, sociology, anthropology, and psychology.

To answer these questions, you will have to draw on your background in social studies, as well as on your ability to understand new material.

In addition to the questions based on reading passages, there are some questions that test your general background knowledge in social studies.

Read the passage through once. Then return to it as often as necessary to answer the questions. *PRINT THE LETTER OF THE CORRECT ANSWER IN THE SPACE AT THE RIGHT.*

Questions 1-5.

DIRECTIONS: Questions 1 through 5 are to be answered on the basis of the following passage.

Over the past several decades, the growth of the United States economy has been marked by expansion of metropolitan areas and by "regionalization" of production—that is, a more even geographical distribution of industries over the United States. Such rapid growth causes drastic changes in the geographical structure of metropolitan areas. Manufacturing industries, which were initially attracted to the core of the city by the proximity of the railroads, a steady labor supply, and the economic advantages of mass production, are now moving toward peripheral locations.

No single explanation can be given for this trend toward suburbanization, but as cities have grown, the supply of undeveloped land has decreased. The advantages of the central metropolis continue to attract economic activity, but congestion in the central city and the development of production techniques which demand more space have tended to push industry into the suburbs. The net result has been a pattern of geographical specialization within metropolitan regions. The central city increasingly becomes geared to white-collar and service activities, and the periphery attracts manufacturing, transportation, and other blue-collar job activities.

The development of residential areas has followed industrial movement to some extent, but suburban living (undoubtedly desired for its amenities) is still largely reserved for those who can afford it. Consequently, the central city has been losing middle- and upper-income families to the suburbs. Now people can live in dispersed residential locations; rising incomes and the proliferation of automobiles have made this both economically and technically feasible. However, this "urban sprawl" creates serious financial problems. Since tax-paying industry has fled to the suburbs, the central city has had to bear the cost of public assistance payments and other welfare service for low-income groups.

When housing developers began building on a large scale, many suburbs rapidly doubled and tripled in size. This new population required more schools and teachers, more fire and police protection, and sizable expenditures for water and sewer lines and roads. Frequently, these towns were entirely dependent on property taxes for their revenues.

To meet ever-increasing expenses and broaden their tax base, some communities have tried to attract new industry. However, when town officials found themselves competing intensely for these industries, they often conceded partial exemption from property taxes to new industry in order to bargain more favorably. As a result, an area often found its tax base weakened rather than strengthened by winning new industry. As a consequence of all these changes, both the suburbs and the central city are entangled in thorny financial problems.

1. According to the author, a rise in wages earned by employees of service industries will PRINCIPALLY tend to
   A. *increase* the physical separation between zones of residence and zones of work
   B. *decrease* the tax revenues of the suburbs
   C. *decrease* the tax revenues of the metropolitan areas
   D. *increase* the work force in the periphery

2. The MOST efficient way to solve the financial problems of a metropolitan area would be to
   A. *cut* personal taxes in central cities
   B. *cut* personal taxes in the suburbs
   C. *decrease* public expenditures in central cities
   D. *place* the entire area under one fiscal authority

3. Which of the following problems should be given FIRST consideration on the basis of the changing urban structure outlined in the passage?
   A. Commuter traffic between areas of residence and areas of work
   B. Highway passenger traffic between two metropolitan areas
   C. Congestion due to heavy truck traffic in downtown areas
   D. The centralization of railroad freight stations in downtown areas

4. The author would consider the giant modern city *essentially* a by-product of the
   A. invention of the internal combustion engine
   B. development of monopolistic industries
   C. Industrial Revolution
   D. capitalist system

5. If the trend outlined in paragraph three continues, the centers of large American cities are more likely than the suburbs to have a HIGH percentage of
   A. small-scale manufacturing firms   B. large-scale factories
   C. railroad stations   D. banks and insurance companies

Questions 6-9.

DIRECTIONS: Questions 6 through 9 are to be answered on the basis of the following passage.

(In 1845, congressional leaders debated the annexation of Texas. The issues considered were many and complex, as the following excerpts from the debate illustrate.)

Speaker 1:
　　In annexing Texas, we do not adopt its war with Mexico, if any such exists. In annexation, we will not abide by Texas law; Texas will abide by ours. The United States are not to be merged in Texas, but Texas in them. When we purchased Louisiana from France, France was at war; we did not assume the French war. Mexico, however, may regard annexation as an act of extreme unfriendliness and make it the pretext for declaring war on the United States.

Speaker 2:
　　Since the landing of the Pilgrims, our people have moved forward, acquiring territory, unfurling the banner of liberty and equality, creating a power (more potent than that of armies), before which the nations of this continent will continue to give way. No nation can withstand the impact of this principle of enlightened liberty. Under this principle—though I regret to say, sometimes backed by the sword—we have been a progressive, but peaceful, people.

Speaker 3:
　　The Anglo-Saxon race, like a mighty flood, has swept over the continent. Some say the flood ought to stop at the Del Norte. I can tell them that it will not. In fifty years it will cover Mexico; in a hundred, Argentina.

Speaker 4:
　　The question of admitting Texas seems to make many apprehensive about the balance of political power. Let them look at the complexion of the House. Let them look also at the map and see the broad expanse of land in the north and northwest which is yet to be made into states where slavery can never exist. In addition, by rejecting Texas, we ensure the spread of slavery. Admit Texas, and the Rio Bravo constitutes the limits of this institution. Reject her, and slavery will not stop until its standard waves in triumph over Mexico.

Speaker 5:
　　Those who advocate annexation contend that the federal government is one of limited powers. Yet they ask that Congress assume the important power of adding a foreign nation to our own. We are referred to the provision in the Constitution that authorizes Congress to admit new states. History shows that this clause was intended only to confer on Congress the power of admitting new states created from territory already belonging to the United States.

Speaker 6:
　　This is the true cause of most of the opposition: fear that an influence opposed to the interests of the manufacturers would be added to the national councils. —

6. Which speaker's argument seems to stem DIRECTLY from a belief in the inevitability of historical events?　　　　1.____
　　A. 5　　　　　　B. 4　　　　　　C. 3　　　　　　D. 1

7. Which of the following is TRUE of Speaker 2's description of the United States' method of acquiring new territory as *peaceful*?
   It
   A. is contradicted by other parts of his statement
   B. is supported by U.S. success in acquiring territories
   C. supports a Marxist interpretation of history
   D. is an accurate but unsupported statement

8. What EARLIER action of Congress was based on the principle of *balance of power* to which Speaker 4 refers?
   The
   A. Northwest Ordinance
   B. Judiciary Act
   C. Missouri Compromise
   D. Great Compromise

9. The argument of which speaker implies that United States territory should be limited to that acquired by an agreement?
   A. 5
   B. 3
   C. 2
   D. 1

Questions 10-15.

DIRECTIONS: Questions 10 through 15 are NOT based on a reading passage. You are to answer these questions on the basis of your background in social studies.

10. Andrew Jackson's term as President is noteworthy LARGELY because during that period
    A. peaceful relations were established with the Plains Indians
    B. the common man came too have more of a say in government
    C. a national bank was established, resulting in this country's first stable currency
    D. women received the right to vote for the first time

11. The 80-day injunction provision of the Taft-Hartley Act was included for what purpose?
    To
    A. provide a cooling-off period allowing labor and management additional time to resolve disputes
    B. permit the unions to arrange for a survey of membership opinion regarding a strike
    C. permit management to update the profit-loss picture for the forthcoming quarter
    D. give government negotiators the time to make a decision about whether a strike would be advisable

12. Which of the following might anthropologists find SIMILAR in purpose to the rain dance of the Pueblo Indians?
    A. The playing of the national anthem before sporting events
    B. Traditional country folk dancing
    C. Studies carried out by a college of agriculture to improve the yield of wheat
    D. A prayer meeting in an American church

13. The MOST significant advance of the Charter of the United Nations over the Covenant of the League of Nations is the
    A. article providing for an international police force to prevent aggression
    B. provision granting veto power to the five permanent members of the Security Council
    C. belief in the maintenance of world peace by international cooperation
    D. establishment of a council with authority to formulate plans for the reduction of armaments

14. The MAIN purpose of the Bill of Rights is to
    A. prevent presidents from telling states what to do
    B. enlarge the scope of the powers of the federal government
    C. reduce the power of the Supreme Court to declare acts of Congress unconstitutional
    D. limit the power of the federal government to abuse individual freedom

15. When Western Europe was cut off from some of its Middle Eastern oil by the Suez crisis in 1956, MOST of the petroleum deficit was made up by the United States and
    A. Canada
    B. Eastern Europe
    C. Indonesia
    D. Venezuela

KEY (CORRECT ANSWERS)

1. A	6. C	11. A
2. D	7. A	12. D
3. A	8. C	13. A
4. C	9. A	14. D
5. D	10. B	15. D

TEST 4

NATURAL SCIENCES READING

DIRECTIONS: This test measures your ability to understand, analyze, and evaluate passages on scientific topics and descriptions of experiments in such fields as biology, chemistry, physics, and physical science.

To answer these questions, you will have to draw on your scientific background as well as on your ability to understand new material.

In addition to the questions based on reading passages, there are some questions that test your general background knowledge in the sciences.

Read the passage through once. Then return to it as often as necessary to answer the questions. *PRINT THE LETTER OF THE CORRECT ANSWER IN THE SPACE AT THE RIGHT.*

Questions 1-5.

DIRECTIONS: Questions 1 through 5 are to be answered on the basis of the following passage.

As the cells that make up different tissues and organs differ in structure and function, so also do they differ in their response to radiation. The law of Bergonie and Tribondeau states that the radiosensitivity of a tissue is directly proportional to its reproductive capacity and inversely proportional to its degree of specialization. In other words, immature, rapidly-dividing cells will be most harmed by radiation. In addition, three other factors are important: undernourished cells are less sensitive than normal ones, the higher the metabolic rate in a cell the lower its resistance to radiation and cells are more sensitive to radiation at specific stages of division.

Radiation alters the electrical charges of the atoms in the irradiated material, breaking the valence bonds holding the molecules together. For example, radiation passing through a cell is most likely to strike water molecules. The breakdown products from these molecules may combine with oxygen to form bleaches, which in turn can break down protein molecules in the cell. One class of these proteins comprises the enzymes that not only play a role in nearly all biochemical reactions but also control cell division. Such inhibition of cell division may permit cells to grow to an abnormal size; when such a cell dies, there is no replacement to fill the void in the tissue. If the cell has been altered so that its daughter cells are genetically different from the parent cell, the daughter cells may die before they reproduce themselves; they may continue to grow without dividing or they may divide at a higher or lower rate than the parent cell.

Because of these possible effects, doctors and scientists have been concerned about the exposure of humans to radiation. A study of the effects of radiation on the human body indicates that the following organ and tissue groups are most affected by radioactivity: (1) blood and bone marrow, (2) lymphatic system, (3) skin and hair follicles, (4) alimentary canal, (5) adrenal glands, (6) thyroid gland, (7.) lungs, (8) urinary tract, (9) liver and gallbladder, (10) bone,

(11) eyes, and (12) reproductive organs. Although no permissible level for exposure of humans to radiation has been established, data reported in 1957 indicate that 25 roentgens cause no observable reaction, 50 roentgens produce nausea and vomiting, 400 to 500 roentgens give the individual a fifty-fifty chance of survival without medical care, and 650 roentgens are lethal.

1. In the first paragraph, the metabolic rate of a cell refers to the cell's
    A. chemical activities
    B. degree of specialization
    C. stage of division
    D. maturity

2. Why is muscle tissue relatively unaffected by radiation? It(s)
    A. cells contain no water
    B. is highly specialized
    C. is protected by the bony skeleton
    D. cells have a unique method of reproduction

3. If radiation can cause cancer as implied in the second paragraph, then which of the following BEST justifies the use of radiation in treating cancer?
    A. Cancer tissue is highly specialized, hence very sensitive to radiation.
    B. Only the cancer cells receive the radiation.
    C. Cancer cells divide relatively rapidly.
    D. The patient may die anyway, and desperate measures are appropriate in such instances.

4. Which of the following would the author probably consider the MOST serious long-range effect of exposure to radiation on human populations?
    A. Possible destruction of natural resources essential to survival
    B. Hereditary changes that might occur in the population
    C. The world's population increasing at a higher rate than the world's food supply
    D. The daughters of people exposed to radiation dying before they can have children

5. Why would a man in outer space be in GREATER danger from radiation than a man on earth?
    A. He would not be shielded from cosmic rays by the earth's atmosphere.
    B. The reduced pressure in a space vehicle inhibits cell division.
    C. Biochemical reactions essential to life cannot occur in outer space.
    D. In a weightless condition, cells are more vulnerable to radiation.

Questions 6-9.

DIRECTIONS: Questions 6 through 9 are to be answered on the basis of the following passage.

A series of experiments was designed to determine how bats are able to fly at night without colliding with obstacles. Bats were released in a closed room across which were strung fine wires adapted to register every time they were touched by one of the bats. The bats were released in the room under the following conditions:

Experiment 1:
The room was well illuminated.

Experiment 2:
The room was completely darkened.

Experiment 3:
The room was darkened, and the bats' eyes were sealed with soft black wax.

Experiment 4:
The room was darkened, the bats' eyes were waxed closed, and numerous small radar transmitters were set in operation throughout the room.

Experiment 5:
The radar transmitters were replaced with loudspeakers which emitted high-frequency sound waves. The room was dark, and the bats' eyes were waxed closed.

Experiment 6:
The lights were turned on, and the bats, without wax on their eyes, were released while the loudspeakers were still producing high-frequency sounds.

On the basis of these experiments, the following observations were made:

In Experiments 1 through 4, the bats did not collide with the wires.

In Experiment 5, the bats seemed confused and frequently collided with the wires.

In Experiment 6, the bats were initially confused and collided with the wires; however, the number of collisions soon decreased.

6. Which conclusion, if any, can be drawn from Experiment 1? 6.____
   A. Bats need light to see where they are going.
   B. Bats need sound waves in order to avoid obstacles.
   C. Bats can see in the dark.
   D. None of the above

7. Which conclusion, if any, can be drawn from Experiment 4? 7.____
   A. Bats evidently use some sort of radar to guide themselves.
   B. The presence of radar waves has no apparent effect on the bats.
   C. The presence of radar waves confuses the bats by obstructing their natural means of locating obstacles.
   D. None of the above

8. Which experiment or group of experiments listed below shows that bats can ordinarily fly safely without using their eyes? 8.____
   A. 3 only   B. 1 and 2   C. 1 and 3   D. 1, 2, 3

9. Which of the following is TRUE about the statement: *Bats are nocturnal animals because daylight interferes with their ability to avoid obstacles.*
   The statement
   A. agrees with the data
   B. is contradicted by the data
   C. cannot be judged without more data
   D. is an experimental assumption

Questions 10-13.

DIRECTIONS: Questions 10 through 13 are NOT based on a reading passage. You are to answer these questions on the basis of your background in the natural sciences.

10. The emergence of new strains of houseflies capable of withstanding the poisonous effects of the chemical DDT is an example of
    A. adaptation   B. the Mendelian law
    C. implementation   D. regeneration

11. What is the MAIN difference between a gas and a liquid?
    A. Molecular weight
    B. Shape of the particles
    C. Geometric arrangement of the molecules
    D. Average distance between the molecules

12. How were the coral reefs of tropical seas formed? By
    A. the accumulation of the remains of small marine animals
    B. the erosion of islands by wind and sea
    C. the accumulation of salts and minerals precipitated by the sea
    D. undersea earthquakes

13. A warm breeze may seem cool to a bather who has just come out of the water because
    A. water is a good conductor of heat
    B. moisture from the air condenses on the skin and cools it
    C. the evaporation of water from the wet skin absorbs heat
    D. water is denser than air

KEY (CORRECT ANSWERS)

1.	A	6.	D	11.	D
2.	B	7.	B	12.	A
3.	C	8.	A	13.	C
4.	B	9.	B		
5.	A	10.	A		

EXAMINATION SECTION
TEST 1

DIRECTIONS: Each question or incomplete statement is followed by several suggested answers or completions. Select the one that BEST answers the question or completes the statement. *PRINT THE LETTER OF THE CORRECT ANSWER IN THE SPACE AT THE RIGHT.*

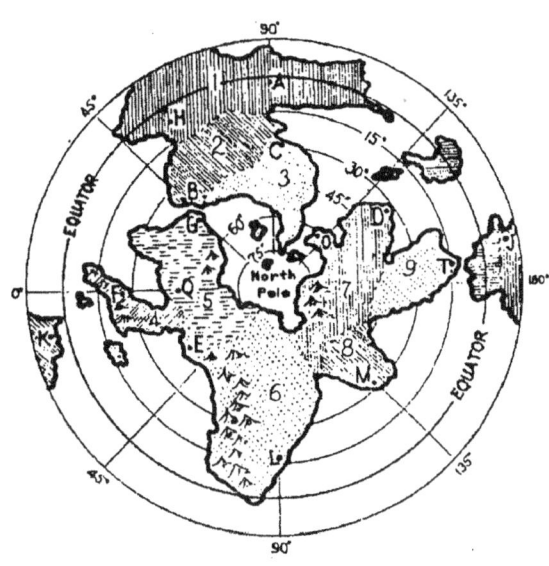

Questions 1-10.

DIRECTIONS: Questions 1-10 are based upon the map above. This map represents a hypothetical planet of the same size as the Earth and occupying the same relative position in a solar system identical with ours. It is supposedly governed by the same physical laws and experiences the same climatic conditions as the Earth.

1. An important advantage of this projection is that 1.____

   A. shapes are not distorted
   B. a single scale of miles may be used
   C. it resembles most nearly the shape of the Earth
   D. it is easier to read than other types
   E. it shows the shortest route between any two places in the North Temperate Zone as an approximately straight line

2. Which of these countries probably has the widest variation in climatic conditions? 2.____

   A. 1   B. 6   C. 7   D. 9   E. 5

3. Which of these cities is farthest south? 3.____

   A. A   B. B   C. C   D. F   E. L

23

4. What is the *approximate* location of city D?

   A. Long. 150° W lat. 30° N
   B. Long 150° W lat. 30° S
   C. Long 30° N lat. 150° E
   D. Long. 30° N lat. 150° W
   E. Long. 150° E lat. 30° S

5. A great circle route from city C to city M would pass *approximately* through

   A. D
   B. G
   C. O
   D. T
   E. the North Pole

6. A storm experienced at city Q would probably have been experienced earlier at

   A. E
   B. G
   C. H
   D. K
   E. the North Pole

7. The SHORTEST route between which two cities crosses the South Pole?

   A. A and J
   B. B and M
   C. D and E
   D. D and L
   E. J and K

8. In which direction is city D from city M?

   A. North
   B. East
   C. West
   D. Northeast
   E. Southwest

9. A plant placed in a window of a house in city K in June would receive MOST sunlight if the window faced

   A. north
   B. east
   C. south
   D. west
   E. impossible to tell

10. Which of these cities is strategically located on the oceanic trade route from D to E?

    A. G   B. K   C. M   D. O   E. T

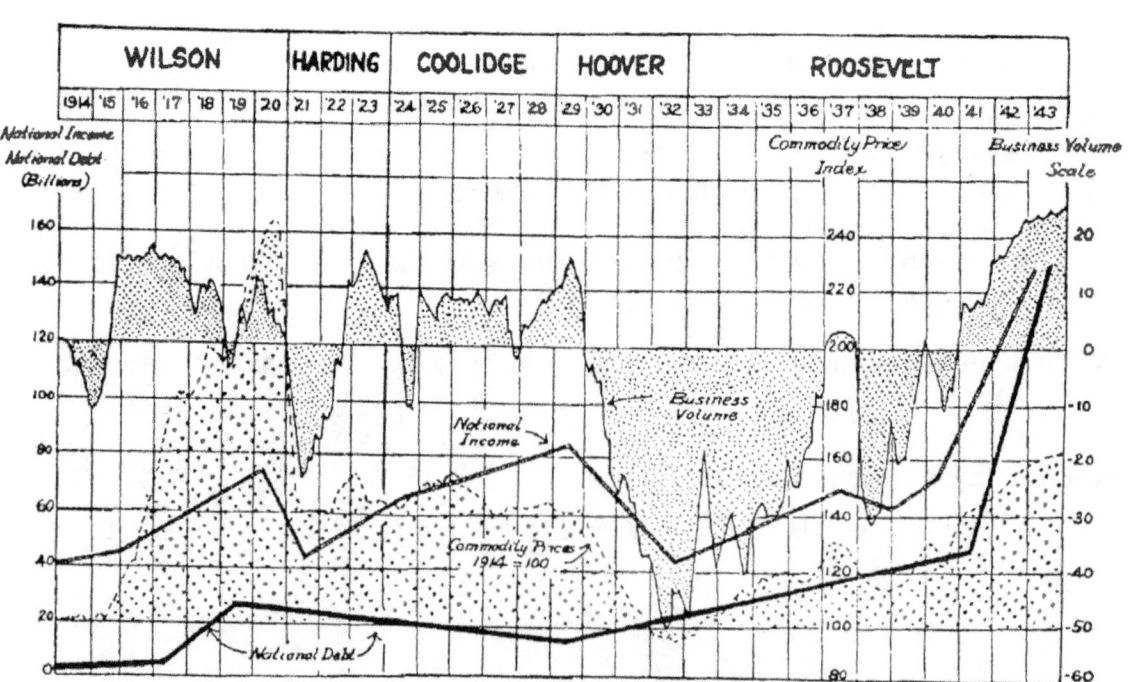

Questions 11-20.

DIRECTIONS: In Questions 11-20, select the alternatives that MOST satisfactorily complete the statements or answer the questions, basing your choice on information given in the chart above or *on your understanding of the economic history of the United States.*

11. As used in the chart, the term *national debt* means the TOTAL amount owned by   11.____

   A. the United States Government to other nations
   B. the federal government
   C. the federal and state governments to United States citizens
   D. the United States Government and United States citizens to foreign persons or nations
   E. United States citizens to other nations

12. Which of the following statements about the national debt of the United States are *true*?   12.____
   I. It increased sharply during both World Wars.
   II. It increased throughout the great depression.
   III. It decreased a third between World War I and the stock market crash.
   IV. In 1943 it had reached the highest point up to that time.
   The CORRECT combination is:

   A. I, II   B. I, III   C. I, IV
   D. III, IV   E. *All* of them

13. As used in the chart, the term *national income* means the   13.____

   A. total of the incomes subject to the federal income tax
   B. value of the goods produced and services rendered in the United States
   C. value of goods and services exported
   D. total of all government revenues in the United States
   E. total revenues of the federal government from taxes and borrowing

14. Which of the following statements about the national income of the United States are *true*?   14.____
   I. It reached its highest point in the period between the declaration of World War I and the declaration of World War II.
   II. It increased constantly after Franklin D. Roosevelt became President.
   III. It increased more in Republican than in Democratic administrations.
   The CORRECT combination is:

   A. *None* of them   B. I *only*   C. I, II
   D. I, III   E. II, III

15. The cost of living   15.____

   A. depends exclusively upon the demand for and the supply of goods
   B. is computed for this chart on the basis of the price level of 1937
   C. is higher in depressions than in normal times
   D. varies inversely with the purchasing power of money
   E. normally decreases when the amount of money in circulation increases

16. As shown by the chart, the index of the cost of living in the United States
    I. is based upon commodity prices in 1914
    II. rose by approximately the same rate in both wars
    III. remained fairly constant throughout the administrations of Harding and Coolidge
    IV. reached a maximum of 165 during World War I
    The CORRECT combination is:

    A. I, II   B. I, III   C. I, IV
    D. II, III   E. II, IV

17. The volume of business

    A. is dependent upon the political party in power
    B. reflects changes in the national debt
    C. is measured by various indexes or "business barometers"
    D. has little relation to prosperity and depression
    E. depends chiefly upon the current tariff policy

18. Which of the following statements about the volume of business in the United States are true?
    I. It has fluctuated widely in the period covered by the chart.
    II. It has shown the same general trends as the national income.
    III. In the period shown, it has been both highest and lowest under Republican Presidents.
    IV. It tends to increase in wartime.
    The CORRECT combination is:

    A. I, II, III   B. I, II, IV   C. I, III, IV
    D. II, III, IV   E. All of them

19. Temporary fluctuations in the value of money depend PRIMARILY on the

    A. cost of food
    B. backing for the money
    C. national income
    D. volume of business in the country
    E. relation between the amount of money and credit and the volume of business

20. In the period shown, which of the following statements about the value of money in the United States are true?
    I. It was greatest at the end of 1932.
    II. It has shown an upward trend during the New Deal.
    III. It rose sharply with the adoption of the Federal Reserve System.
    IV. It remained higher in the present war than in World War I.
    The CORRECT combination is:

    A. I, II   B. I, IV   C. II, III
    D. II, IV   E. III, IV

21. Within its borders a state controls all of the following EXCEPT

    A. qualifications for voting   B. chartering of corporations
    C. naturalization of aliens   D. the insurance business
    E. conduct of elections

22. The Federal Government was empowered to regulate interstate and foreign commerce by a(n)

    A. law passed by Congress
    B. provision in the Federal Constitution
    C. compromise between Hamilton and Jefferson
    D. Supreme Court decision
    E. amendment to the Federal Constitution

22.____

23. Jefferson claimed that his purchase of the Louisiana Territory was constitutional because of the

    A. treaty-making clause
    B. power to regulate foreign and interstate commerce
    C. clause relating to general welfare
    D. President's powers as commander in chief of the Army and Navy
    E. power to execute the laws

23.____

24. Sources from which Hamilton received the LARGEST amount of revenue were

    A. land tax and dividends from the first United States Bank
    B. tariff and land taxes
    C. excise and land taxes
    D. excise and income taxes
    E. tariff and excise taxes

24.____

25. In the first decade of the 19th century, the route by which it was *cheapest* for a farmer in the southern part of Illinois to ship his produce to a seaport was by the

    A. Missouri and Mississippi Rivers
    B. Great Lakes and the Erie Canal
    C. Baltimore and Ohio Railroad
    D. Ohio and Mississippi Rivers
    E. Cumberland Road

25.____

26. The author who urged American writers and artists to use the American scene in their creations rather than to imitate European models and is said to have stated America's "intellectual declaration of independence" was

    A. Washington Irving   B. Nathaniel Hawthorne
    C. Ralph Waldo Emerson   D. James Russell Lowell
    E. Thomas Jefferson

26.____

27. What famous American inventor has attained *posthumous* recognition for his ability in art?

    A. Joseph Henry   B. Cyrus McCormick
    C. Samuel F. B. Morse   D. Elmer Sperry
    E. Eli Whitney

27.____

28. Of the following factors, the one that was MOST influential in bringing about the rise of the factory system in the United States was

   A. the invention of the sewing machine
   B. Washington's proclamation of neutrality
   C. the establishment of the first United States Bank
   D. the tariff act of 1789
   E. the Napoleonic Wars

29. Before the Civil War, wages in the United States were *higher* than in European countries because

   A. the cost of living was higher
   B. immigration was restricted
   C. labor was scarce in comparison to the resources to be developed
   D. labor unions had demanded them
   E. there was a high protective tariff

30. At the outbreak of the Civil War, the *major* railroad lines in the United States

   A. were found chiefly in New England
   B. had reached the Rocky Mountains
   C. ran north and south in the eastern half of the country
   D. were located chiefly in the North, running west to the Mississippi Valley
   E. extended to the Pacific

KEY (CORRECT ANSWERS)

1.	E	16.	B
2.	B	17.	C
3.	A	18.	B
4.	A	19.	E
5.	C	20.	B
6.	B	21.	C
7.	E	22.	B
8.	B	23.	A
9.	A	24.	E
10.	E	25.	D
11.	B	26.	C
12.	E	27.	C
13.	B	28.	E
14.	A	29.	C
15.	D	30.	D

TEST 2

DIRECTIONS: Each question or incomplete statement is followed by several suggested answers or completions. Select the one that BEST answers the question or completes the statement. *PRINT THE LETTER OF THE CORRECT ANSWER IN THE SPACE AT THE RIGHT.*

1. Important planks in the platform of the Republican party in 1860 were   1.____

    A. exclusion of slavery from the territories, a homestead law, protective tariff
    B. free territories, income tax, protective tariff
    C. abolition of slavery, manifest destiny, popular election of United States Senators
    D. abolition of the slave trade, excise taxes, regulation of railroads
    E. exclusion of slavery from the territories, purchase of Alaska, reciprocal tariffs

2. *Before* 1860, the currency of the United States was based on   2.____

    A. a managed dollar
    B. the gold standard
    C. a silver standard
    D. a gold bullion standard
    E. a bimetallic standard

3. The clause of the Federal Constitution MOST liberally interpreted by President Lincoln was that giving the President power to   3.____

    A. make recess appointments
    B. make treaties
    C. raise an army
    D. coin money and regulate its value
    E. act as commander in chief of the Army and Navy

4. The greenbacks issued during the Civil War   4.____

    A. stabilized prices
    B. increased the cost of the war
    C. increased the prosperity of the professional groups
    D. caused gold to circulate more freely
    E. lowered the prices of farm products

5. The MAJOR purpose of the Morrill Act (1862) and the Hatch Act (1887) was to provide funds for   5.____

    A. education of the Indians
    B. training teachers of higher education
    C. education of seamen
    D. training engineers
    E. scientific farming

6. In 1894, the Supreme Court declared the federal income tax unconstitutional because it   6.____

    A. was not apportioned according to population
    B. interfered with the right of states to fix incomes
    C. was a form of double taxation
    D. was an indirect tax
    E. was not uniform throughout the country

29

7. The Hague Conferences of 1899 and 1907 did NOT

   A. provide for an international prize court
   B. provide for more humane warfare
   C. indorse the "Drago doctrine"
   D. set up machinery for settling international disputes
   E. reduce armaments

8. The Five-Power Treaty of the Washington Conference in 1922 provided for the

   A. settlement of all disputes by arbitration
   B. territorial integrity of China
   C. limitation of naval armaments
   D. protection of South America
   E. acceptance of the Stimson Doctrine

9. A method of payment of war debts from World War I was provided for in the

   A. Root formula   B. Johnson Act   C. Stimson note
   D. Young Plan   E. Lytton Report

10. In the 20th century, farmers have NOT demanded

    A. a moratorium on farm-mortgage foreclosures
    B. draft deferment of farm workers
    C. government-owned grain elevators
    D. crop insurance
    E. application of antitrust legislation to farming

11. A reason for the construction of dams in many areas of the United States that was of *little* importance in the Tennessee Valley development was the

    A. desire to raise living standards
    B. need for irrigation
    C. desire to develop water power
    D. need to prevent erosion
    E. need for flood control

12. The enactment of the Neutrality Law of 1935 was influenced by a Senate investigation of

    A. the sale of scrap iron to Japan
    B. munitions manufacturers
    C. un-American activities
    D. airplane concerns
    E. the oil industry

13. At the outbreak of World War II, the *three* countries that controlled MOST of the land area of the world were

    A. China, France, Great Britain
    B. the United States, France, China
    C. Great Britain, France, the United States
    D. Great Britain, Soviet Union, France
    E. Soviet Union, the United States, Holland

14. The United States Government prefers to sell war bonds to individuals rather than to banks because the					14.____

   A. average person is hoarding his high wartime wages
   B. banks are reluctant to invest large sums of money in such bonds
   C. tendency of such sales is to avert inflation
   D. Administration fears the domination of the Government by the banking interests
   E. Government wants to give its citizens the opportunity for safe investments at high interest rates

15. At the Bretton Woods Conference plans were made about					15.____

   A. postwar aviation   B. a world granary
   C. relief and rehabilitation D. dissolution of cartels
   E. an international bank

16. In the presidential election of 1944, eighteen-year-olds were eligible to vote in					16.____

   A. Georgia   B. Massachusetts   C. Nebraska
   D. California   E. Wyoming

17. An American appointed as a delegate to the conference of the United Nations at San Francisco was					17.____

   A. Clare Boothe Luce   B. Edith Nourse Rogers
   C. Virginia Gildersleeve   D. Mabel Newcomer
   E. Dorothy Thompson

18. The procedure of allowing a bill to become a law without the President's signature was followed by					18.____

   A. Lincoln on the National Banking Act
   B. Cleveland on the Wilson-Gorman tariff
   C. Taft on the Payne-Aldrich tariff
   D. Wilson on the Federal Reserve Act
   E. Hoover on the Hawley-Smooth tariff

19. The period since the Civil War has been one of high protective tariffs. A tariff act of this period that brought *considerable* reduction in the general average of tariff rates was the					19.____

   A. McKinley tariff   B. Dingley tariff
   C. Underwood tariff   D. Hawley-Smoot tariff
   E. Fordney-McCumber tariff

20. The "resumption of specie payments" refers to the					20.____

   A. redemption of United States notes in gold
   B. requirement that western lands be paid for in gold
   C. establishment of the gold dollar as the monetary standard of the United States
   D. resumption of normal banking operations after the bank holiday in 1933
   E. resumption after the bank holiday of the settlement of foreign trade balances by the exportation of gold

21. Which of the following candidates for President of the United States was NOT a Governor of New York State?

    A. Grover Cleveland
    B. Charles E. Hughes
    C. William McKinley
    D. Alfred E. Smith
    E. Samuel J. Tilden

22. Under existing legislation, the Board of Governors of the Federal Reserve System can NOT

    A. require reports from member banks at regular intervals
    B. engage in open market operations in United States bonds
    C. establish margin requirements of stock exchange transactions
    D. alter the gold content of the dollar
    E. change the reserve requirements for banks

23. All of the following policies have been advocated generally by organized labor in the United States EXCEPT

    A. government ownership of basic industries
    B. liberal support of free public education
    C. voting by union members in political elections for candidates who favor labor
    D. restricted immigration
    E. the closed shop

24. Which of the following statements about industrial unions is NOT true? They

    A. grew up largely in mass-production industries
    B. form a majority group of the AFL-CIO
    C. are made up of both skilled and unskilled workers
    D. are trade associations
    E. are vertical unions

25. All of the following are labor organizations EXCEPT the

    A. Order of Sleeping Car Conductors
    B. American Federation of Musicians
    C. American Newspaper Guild
    D. National Maritime Union
    E. Consumers' Union

26. All of the following practices formerly used by employers are now illegal EXCEPT the

    A. giving of financial assistance to a union
    B. company-sponsored pension system
    C. bringing of strikebreakers across state lines
    D. yellow-dog contract
    E. blacklist

27. In most states, compensation insurance

    A. is subsidized by the State Government
    B. is required of all employers
    C. covers employes engaged in intrastate production only
    D. is required only in certain dangerous industries
    E. is paid for by the employer

28. The pioneer countries in the movement for accident, sickness, unemployment and old-age insurance were

    A. Germany and the United States
    B. the United States and England
    C. New Zealand and France
    D. Denmark and Russia
    E. Germany and New Zealand

28.____

29. In the United States, the social-security program

    A. served as a model for the Beveridge Plan
    B. provides unemployment insurance for all workers
    C. is administered entirely by the Federal Government
    D. supports its old-age insurance feature by a payroll tax on both employers and employes
    E. requires workers to retire at the age of 60

29.____

30. In order to obtain a social-security number, the worker must

    A. be at least 16 years of age
    B. be engaged in an occupation not specifically exempted
    C. get a salary of at least $12 a week
    D. have evidence of United States citizenship
    E. have an application signed by a parent

30.____

KEY (CORRECT ANSWERS)

1.	A	16.	A
2.	E	17.	C
3.	E	18.	E
4.	B	19.	C
5.	E	20.	A
6.	A	21.	C
7.	E	22.	D
8.	C	23.	A
9.	D	24.	D
10.	E	25.	E
11.	B	26.	B
12.	B	27.	E
13.	D	28.	E
14.	C	29.	D
15.	E	30.	B

TEST 3

Questions 1-30.

DIRECTIONS: In Questions 1-30, the possible answers are numbered I, II, III, IV, V. *Any, all* or *none* of these answers may be right. In each case choose from the alternatives lettered A to E the one that includes the numbers preceding *all* the right answers. *PRINT THE LETTER OF THE CORRECT ANSWER IN THE SPACE AT THE RIGHT.*

1. Which of these quotations are from the Declaration of Independence?
    I. "All men are created equal"
    II. "Congress shall make no law respecting an establishment of religion–"
    III. "A government of the people, by the people, for the people"
    IV. "Governments are instituted among men, deriving their just powers from the consent of the governed"

    The CORRECT combination is:

    A. I, II, III   B. I, III   C. I, III, IV
    D. I, IV   E. III, IV

    1.___

2. By which of the following may powers granted by the Constitution be extended?
    I. Federal legislation
    II. Custom
    III. Court interpretations
    IV. Formal amendment

    The CORRECT combination is:

    A. I, II, IV   B. I, III   C. I, IV
    D. IV *only*   E. *All* of them

    2.___

3. Which of the following statements about the Louisiana Purchase are *true*?
    I. It gave the United States control of the Mississippi River.
    II. It removed Spain as the western neighbor of the United States.
    III. It established the Mississippi as the western boundary of the United States.
    IV. It violated the doctrine of isolation.
    V. It set a precedent for allowing the future acquisition of territories by the United States.

    The CORRECT combination is:

    A. I, II, IV   B. I, IV   C. I, V
    D. II, III, IV   E. *All* of them

    3.___

4. Nation-wide organizations in the United States attempted during the 19th century to influence public opinion concerning
    I. abolition of slavery
    II. woman's rights
    III. temperance
    IV. shorter working day
    V. world peace

    The CORRECT combination is:

    A. I, II, III, IV   B. II, III, IV, V   C. II, V
    D. III, IV, V   E. *All* of them

    4.___

34

5. Which of the following statements concerning education are *true* for the period before the Civil War?
   I. Most students preparing to enter college attended private academies.
   II. There were only two colleges or universities that received their chief support from state revenue.
   III. Most medical colleges placed little emphasis on laboratory and clinical training.
   IV. The majority of lawyers had not studied for even a year at a regular law school.
   V. Girls were excluded from most public elementary and secondary schools.
   The CORRECT combination is:

   A. I, III, IV
   B. I, IV, V
   C. II, III, IV
   D. III, IV
   E. III, V

6. Some of the reasons for the establishment of the national banking system in 1863 were the need to
   I. unify the banking system
   II. provide a sounder currency
   III. sell government bonds
   It was *reasonably successful* in accomplishing

   A. *none* of them
   B. I, II
   C. I, III
   D. II, III
   E. *all of* them

7. The Monroe Doctrine would apply to which of the following cases?
   I. England's granting of dominion status to British Guiana
   II. Russian interference in China's political affairs
   III. An attempt by Spain to set up a puppet government in the Argentine
   IV. Japanese interference in the Mexican government
   V. A transfer of the island of Madagascar by France to England
   The CORRECT combination is:

   A. I, III, IV
   B. II, III, V
   C. III, IV
   D. III *only*
   E. IV *only*

8. In which of the following periods did the power of the President show a *great* tendency to increase?
   I. 1816-28
   II. 1829-37
   III. 1884-1900
   IV. 1901-20
   V. 1921-29
   The CORRECT combination is:

   A. *None* of them
   B. I, IV
   C. II, IV
   D. II, V
   E. *All* of them

9. In wartime, governments resort to various means of raising money, among them
    I. issuance of inadequately backed money
    II. issuance and sale of bonds
    III. increase in tariff rates
    IV. sharp increase in taxes
   In *all* of the following wars: the Civil War, First World War and Second World War, the United States Government raised money by

   A. I, II B. I, IV C. II, IV
   D. III, IV E. *all* of them

10. Which of the following panics resulted in banking reform?
    I. 1873
    II. 1893
    III. 1907
    IV. 1929
    The CORRECT combination is:

    A. I, II B. I, IV C. II, III
    D. II, IV E. III, IV

11. In which of the following fields did state legislation *precede* national legislation?
    I. Regulation of the railroads
    II. Abolition of child labor
    III. Popular election of United States Senators
    IV. Better housing
    V. Woman suffrage
    The CORRECT combination is:

    A. I, II, IV, V B. II, III, IV, V C. II, IV
    D. II, IV, V E. *All of* them

12. Which of the following statements about Pan-Americanism are *true*?
    I. Henry Clay advocated that the United States recognize the independence of the Latin-American States.
    II. In 1889 Simon Bolivar called the Pan-American Conference which organized the first Pan-American Union.
    III. The Pan-American movement was known as the Pan-Hispanic movement until Canada became a member.
    IV. The relation of Pan-Americanism to world organization was given consideration at the Mexico City Conference of 1945.
    V. Argentina declared war on the Axis after the Mexico City Conference of 1945.
    The CORRECT combination is:

    A. I, II, IV B. I, IV C. I, IV, V
    D. II, III, V E. IV, V

13. Which *two* of the following quotations express the *strongest* national feeling? 13.____
    I. "The Union, next to our liberty, the most dear." - Calhoun
    II. "I have heard something said about allegiance to the South. I know no South, no North, no East, no West, to which I owe any allegiance." - Clay
    III. "I have no unseemly comment to offer on the league of Nations. But it is not for us." - *Harding*
    IV. "You have not conquered the South. You never will ... The war for the Union is, in your hands, a most bloody and costly failure." - *Vallandigham*
    The CORRECT combination is:

    A. I, II   B. I, III   C. I, IV
    D. II, III   E. II, IV

14. Which of the following statements about amusements are *true*? 14.____
    I. The Puritans frowned on amusements and enjoyment of leisure.
    II. Bowling was a popular sport among the Dutch in New Netherland.
    III. Cooperstown is the birthplace of the national game of baseball.
    IV. Most Americans are spectators rather than participants in games and amusements.
    The CORRECT combination is:

    A. I, II   B. I, II, IV   C. II, III, IV
    D. III, IV   E. *All* of them

15. Which of the following statements concerning American architecture are *true*? 15.____
    I. Recent American architecture has shown an increasing tendency to recognize the importance of functionalism.
    II. Thomas Jefferson fostered the revival of the classical influence in architecture in America during the early 1800's.
    III. Within recent years, many newly constructed American churches have followed the Gothic pattern.
    IV. America borrowed the skyscraper type of architecture from Germany and adapted it to American conditions.
    V. Ralph Adams Cram was an advocate of Romanesque architecture.
    The CORRECT combination is:

    A. I, II, III   B. I, II, IV   C. I, IV
    D. II, III, V   E. *All of* them

16. Which of the following statements about schools are *true*? 16.____
    I. Laws prohibiting child labor increase school attendance.
    II. American high school education has been free to all since colonial times.
    III. School district control has been an outstanding example of democratic government.
    IV. The Ordinance of 1787 provided for free compulsory education.
    The CORRECT combination is:

    A. I, II   B. I, II, III   C. I, III
    D. I, IV   E. III, IV

17. Which of the following statements are *true*?
    I. In the United States outstanding advancement has been made in short story writing.
    II. Interpretative dancing is a typically American art.
    III. Only one American writer has been awarded the Nobel prize in literature.
    IV. An original contribution of the United States to music is the Negro spiritual.
    The CORRECT combination is:

    A. I, II, IV   B. I, IV   C. II, III
    D. II, III, IV   E. *All* of them

18. Of the following books, which have MOST directly influenced American history?
    I. THE CRISIS by Tom Paine
    II. LIFE ON THE MISSISSIPPI by Mark Twain
    III. THE GENTLEMAN FROM INDIANA by Booth Tarkington
    IV. MAIN STREET by Sinclair Lewis
    V. THE SHAME OF THE CITIES by Lincoln Steffens
    VI. A CENTURY OF DISHONOR by Helen Hunt Jackson
    The CORRECT combination is:

    A. I, II, IV   B. I, III, V   C. I, V, VI
    D. II, III, VI   E. IV, V

19. Which of the following have been used *against* the interests of labor? The
    I. Wagner-Connery Act
    II. Sherman Anti-Trust Act
    III. 14th amendment to the Constitution
    The CORRECT combination is:

    A. *None* of them   B. I, II   C. I, III
    D. II, III   E. *All* of them

20. Which of the following groups are *exempt* from the provisions of the Fair Labor Standards Act (Wages and Hours Act)?
    I. Factory workers
    II. Railroad employes
    III. Agricultural laborers
    IV. Mine workers
    V. Persons in domestic service
    The CORRECT combination is:

    A. I, III, V   B. I, IV   C. II, III, IV
    D. II, V   E. III, V

21. Which of the following are *great circles*?
    I. Any circle drawn on the globe
    II. Any circle bounding the zones
    III. A circle drawn through the North Pole
    IV. The equator
    V. Any circle whose plane passes through the center of the earth
    The CORRECT combination is:

    A. I, IV, V   B. II, III   C. II, IV, V
    D. IV, V   E. *All* of them

22. A *great circle* is used in planning which of the following? 22.____
    I. Ocean routes
    II. Highways
    III. International railroad routes
    IV. Airplane routes
    The CORRECT combination is:

    A. I, II   B. I, III, IV   C. *I*, IV
    D. IV *only*   E. *All* of them

23. Of which of the following did the United States import MORE than 80% of its supply in 1970? 23.____
    I. Tin
    II. Copper
    III. Rubber
    IV. Coal
    V. Oil
    VI. Coffee
    VII. Hemp
    The CORRECT combination is:

    A. I, II, III, V   B. I, III, VI, VII   C. II, III, IV, V, VI
    D. IV, VI   E. *All* of them

24. Which of the following proposals made during World War II had *counterparts* in World War I? 24.____
    I. Provision for an association of nations
    II. Provision for a World Court
    III. Demands for reparations
    IV. Accessions of territory to Poland at the expense of Germany
    The CORRECT combination is:

    A. I, II   B. I, II, IV   C. I, III, IV
    D. II, III, IV   E. *All* of them

25. Which of the following statements are *true* concerning agreements made at the Dumbarton Oaks Conference of October, 1944? 25.____
    I. An association of nations was established.
    II. Complete agreement was reached on how the Security Council should deal with aggressor nations.
    III. All member nations were to have seats on the Security Council.
    IV. The major decisions were to be made by the Assembly.
    V. Only the Big Five were to have seats on the Security Council.
    The CORRECT combination is:

    A. *None* of them   B. I, II   C. I, III
    D. I, IV   E. II, V

26. Which of the following were writers in the field of *political science?*
    I. Aristotle
    II. John Locke
    III. Charles Darwin
    IV. James Madison
    V. Stephen A. Douglas
    The CORRECT combination is:

    A. I, II, III   B. I, II, IV   C. II, III
    D. IV, V   E. *All* of them

27. Which of the following are classified as *historians?*
    I. Carlton Hayes
    II. Benjamin Franklin
    III. Francis Parkman
    IV. Edward Gibbon
    V. Charles Beard
    The CORRECT combination is:

    A. I, II, III   B. I, III, IV   C. I, III, IV, V
    D. II, III, IV, V   E. II, IV, V

28. Which of the following writers made the *welfare of the common people* the subject of their writings?
    I. Charles Dickens
    II. Walter Scott
    III. Victor Hugo
    IV. Edward Bellamy
    V. Alfred Tennyson
    The CORRECT combination is:

    A. I, III, IV   B. I, IV, V   C. I, V
    D. II, III, IV   E. II, III, V

29. Which of the following advocated *colonial expansion* for Great Britain?
    I. Cecil Rhodes
    II. Gladstone
    III. G. B. Shaw
    IV. Disraeli
    The CORRECT combination is:

    A. I, III   B. I, IV   C. II, III
    D. II, IV   E. III, IV

30. Which of the following statements about India are *true?*
    I. It is a dominion of the British Empire.
    II. Its two dominant religious groups are the Hindus and the Moslems.
    III. It has few natural resources.
    IV. Most of the native princes are opposed to complete Indian independence.
    The CORRECT combination is:

    A. I, II   B. II, III, IV   C. II, IV
    D. III, IV   E. *All* of them

KEY (CORRECT ANSWERS)

1.	D	16.	C
2.	E	17.	B
3.	C	18.	C
4.	A	19.	D
5.	A	20.	C
6.	D	21.	D
7.	C	22.	C
8.	C	23.	B
9.	C	24.	E
10.	E	25.	A
11.	A	26.	B
12.	D	27.	C
13.	D	28.	A
14.	E	29.	B
15.	A	30.	C

TEST 4

DIRECTIONS: Each question or incomplete statement is followed by several suggested answers or completions. Select the one that BEST answers the question or completes the statement. *PRINT THE LETTER OF THE CORRECT ANSWER IN THE SPACE AT THE RIGHT.*

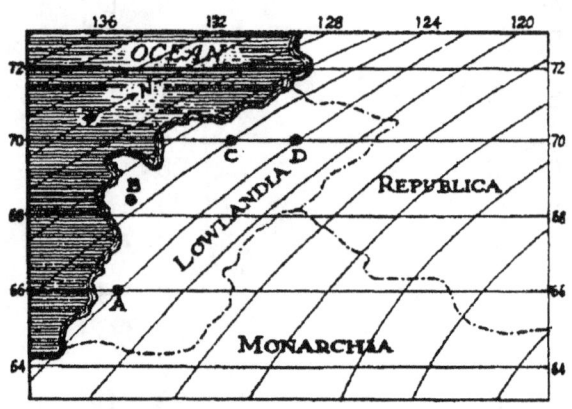

Questions 1-10.

DIRECTIONS: Questions 1-10 inclusive are based upon the map above.

1. The climate of Lowlandia probably *approximates* MOST closely that of   1.___

   A. tundras
   B. wet subtropical areas
   C. marine west coast
   D. rainy low latitudes
   E. continental deserts

2. Assume that in this part of the world no attention is paid to standard time zones and that each city goes by apparent solar time – or sun time. When it is 3:00 p.m. at A, what time is it at C?   2.___

   A. 2:44 p.m.   B. 2:52 p.m.   C. 3:00 p.m.
   D. 3:08 p.m.   E. 3:16 p.m.

3. The distance between A and D is *approximately*   3.___

   A. 7 miles   B. 70 miles   C. 140 miles
   D. 280 miles E. 700 miles

4. Of the following occupations, which would MOST likely be found in this land?   4.___

   A. Cattle ranching   B. Cotton growing
   C. Truck farming   D. Reindeer herding
   E. Tulip growing

5. Lowlandia is located   5.___

   A. north of the equator, east of Greenwich
   B. north of the equator, west of Greenwich
   C. north of the equator, due north of Greenwich
   D. south of the equator, east of Greenwich
   E. south of the equator, west of Greenwich

6. Lowlandia is crossed by the

   A. Arctic Circle
   B. equator
   C. Tropic of Capricorn
   D. Tropic of Cancer
   E. Antarctic Circle

7. The day of the year on which the GREATEST number of hours of daylight are received at D will occur in

   A. June
   B. December
   C. March
   D. September
   E. April

8. On the day of the year on which there is the GREATEST number of hours of daylight, how much daylight do people at D have?

   A. 4 hours
   B. 8 hours
   C. 12 hours
   D. 16 hours
   E. 24 hours

9. Traveling in a straight line from A to B, one would travel

   A. north
   B. northwest
   C. northeast
   D. slightly east of north
   E. slightly west of north

10. If one were to travel due east from A by air, one would eventually reach

    A. Hawaii
    B. British Isles
    C. Australia
    D. Iceland
    E. Newfoundland

KEY (CORRECT ANSWERS)

1. A
2. E
3. D
4. D
5. B
6. A
7. A
8. E
9. E
10. D

WORD MEANING
EXAMINATION SECTION
TEST 1

DIRECTIONS: For the following questions, select the word or group of words lettered A, B, C, D, or E that means MOST NEARLY the same as the word in capital letters. *PRINT THE LETTER OF THE CORRECT ANSWER IN THE SPACE AT THE RIGHT.*

1. The lane was NARROW and led to a mountain lake. 1.____

    A. attractive B. not wide
    C. overgrown D. rough
    E. without trees

2. Blow the horn as you APPROACH the gate. 2.____

    A. discover B. leave
    C. draw near D. pass through
    E. unlock

3. It was part of our BARGAIN that you should wash dishes. 3.____

    A. agreement B. debt C. goal D. plan E. wish

4. I shall remember that little valley FOREVER. 4.____

    A. often B. yet C. always D. next E. no more

5. The boy was EAGER to go on the trip. 5.____

    A. able B. afraid C. anxious D. likely E. willing

6. The children were having a DISPUTE over the boy. 6.____

    A. conversation B. crying spell C. disagreement
    D. performance E. tantrum

7. The man was punished for his BRUTAL act. 7.____

    A. bloody B. cruel
    C. deadly D. defenseless
    E. ugly

8. We LAUNCHED our new business with great hope for the future. 8.____

    A. concluded B. started C. pursued D. steered E. watched

9. The two streets INTERSECT at the edge of town. 9.____

    A. run parallel B. change names C. end
    D. become thoroughfares E. cross

10. She suffered from an UNCOMMON disease. 10.____

    A. ordinary B. painful C. contagious D. rare E. new

45

11. The antique chair was very FRAGILE.

    A. delicate   B. worn   C. beautiful   D. well-made   E. useless

12. They picked EDIBLE mushrooms.

    A. poisonous   B. well-formed   C. unusual   D. large   E. eatable

13. He found the reception at the airport very GRATIFYING.

    A. surprising   B. deafening   C. pleasant
    D. disagreeable   E. impolite

14. DEFECTIVE brakes caused the mishap.

    A. old-fashioned   B. uneven   C. squeaking
    D. unused   E. faulty

15. After a little EXERTION the box was moved.

    A. argument   B. delay   C. coaxing   D. effort   E. planning

KEY (CORRECT ANSWERS)

1. B
2. C
3. A
4. C
5. C

6. C
7. B
8. B
9. E
10. D

11. A
12. E
13. C
14. E
15. D

TEST 2

DIRECTIONS: For the following questions, select the word or group of words lettered A, B, C, D, or E that means MOST NEARLY the same as the word in capital letters. *PRINT THE LETTER OF THE CORRECT ANSWER IN THE SPACE AT THE RIGHT.*

1. The RAPIDITY of the attack surprised us.
   A. power B. effectiveness C. possibility
   D. strangeness E. swiftness

2. She enjoyed CONVERSING with her friends.
   A. meeting B. laughing C. talking D. dining E. traveling

3. There was a small VENT near the end of the tube.
   A. cap B. screw C. opening D. joint E. pump

4. With great CAUTION we opened the barn door.
   A. care B. fear C. distrust D. danger E. difficulty

5. The old man's coat was THREADBARE.
   A. spotted B. tight C. new D. ill-made E. shabby

6. I was sorry that I could not decide OTHERWISE.
   A. immediately B. differently C. favorably
   D. positively E. eagerly

7. The GIGANTIC switchboard controlled all the lights in the theatre.
   A. complicated B. up-to-date C. automatic
   D. huge E. stationary

8. The balls were made of SYNTHETIC rubber.
   A. artificial B. hard C. cheap D. imported E. crude

9. He was MERELY a servant in the house.
   A. occasionally B. in no way C. unhappily
   D. formerly E. no more than

10. The prisoner CONFERRED with his lawyer.
    A. argued B. interfered C. dined
    D. sympathized E. consulted

11. The soldier's GALLANTRY went unnoticed.
    A. strength B. fright
    C. disobedience D. injury
    E. bravery

47

12. The music was chosen for its SOOTHING effect. 12.___
    A. tuneful   B. calming   C. magic   D. exciting   E. solemn
13. The owners were advised to REINFORCE the wall. 13.___
    A. rebuild   B. lengthen   C. lower   D. strengthen   E. repaint
14. They performed their duties with UTMOST ease. 14.___
    A. noticeable   B. some   C. surprising   D. greatest   E. increasing
15. We picnicked near a CASCADE. 15.___
    A. pond   B. camp   C. waterfall   D. trail   E. slope

KEY (CORRECT ANSWERS)

1. E
2. C
3. C
4. A
5. E

6. B
7. D
8. A
9. E
10. E

11. E
12. B
13. D
14. D
15. C

TEST 3

DIRECTIONS: For the following questions, select the word or group of words lettered A, B, C, D, or E that means MOST NEARLY the same as the word in capital letters. *PRINT THE LETTER OF THE CORRECT ANSWER IN THE SPACE AT THE RIGHT.*

1. The chairman was anxious to ADJOURN the meeting.   1.____
   A. conduct   B. attend   C. start   D. address   E. close

2. The gown was made of a GLOSSY fabric.   2.____
   A. shiny   B. embroidered   C. many-colored
   D. transparent   E. expensive

3. An ocean voyage in a small boat can be very HAZARDOUS.   3.____
   A. thrilling   B. slow   C. dangerous   D. rough   E. tiresome

4. The weatherman predicted VARIABLE winds.   4.____
   A. drying   B. strong   C. cool   D. light   E. changeable

5. Not long after the play began, the children began to FIDGET.   5.____
   A. clap   B. move restlessly
   C. cry   D. laugh aloud
   E. shriek

6. That person has a habit of MEDDLING.   6.____
   A. stumbling   B. interfering   C. play jokes
   D. cheating   E. being late

7. Young children are frequently INQUISITIVE.   7.____
   A. curious   B. saucy   C. restless   D. shy   E. tearful

8. The FALSITY of the report was apparent at first glance.   8.____
   A. uselessness   B. untidiness   C. incompleteness
   D. incorrectness   E. disagreeableness

9. Orders were given to LIBERATE the prisoners by noon.   9.____
   A. question   B. transfer   C. free   D. sentence   E. fingerprint

10. She is HABITUALLY late for her dental appointments.   10.____
    A. usually   B. seldom   C. extremely   D. slightly   E. never

11. The soldiers were given SPACIOUS living quarters.   11.____
    A. pleasant   B. well-aired   C. crowded
    D. well-furnished   E. roomy

49

12. The witnesses gave STRAIGHTFORWARD answers.

    A. hasty   B. frank   C. conflicting   D. helpful   E. serious

13. His income EXCEEDS that of his brother.

    A. is less regular than
    B. is greater than
    C. is the same as
    D. is less than
    E. is spent sooner than

14. He SHUNNED all of his neighbors.

    A. disapproved   B. welcomed   C. quarreled with
    D. avoided   E. insulted

15. Many of the natives are ILLITERATE.

    A. unable to read   B. unclean   C. unable to vote
    D. unmanageable   E. sickly

KEY (CORRECT ANSWERS)

1.	E	6.	B
2.	A	7.	A
3.	C	8.	D
4.	E	9.	C
5.	B	10.	A
11.	E		
12.	B		
13.	B		
14.	D		
15.	A		

TEST 4

DIRECTIONS: For the following questions, select the word or group of words lettered A, B, C, D, or E that means MOST NEARLY the same as the word in capital letters. *PRINT THE LETTER OF THE CORRECT ANSWER IN THE SPACE AT THE RIGHT.*

1. We have always found this medicine to be RELIABLE. 1.____
   - A. dependable
   - B. easy to use
   - C. pleasant-tasting
   - D. bitter
   - E. fast-acting

2. The cloth was left to BLEACH in the sun. 2.____
   - A. dry B. soak C. whiten D. shrink E. rot

3. The work is ORDINARILY done on time. 3.____
   - A. seldom
   - B. without fail
   - C. necessarily
   - D. hardly ever
   - E. usually

4. Jim is a very DISCOURTEOUS boy. 4.____
   - A. impolite B. daring C. untruthful D. uneasy E. cautious

5. Paris is noted for its BOULEVARDS. 5.____
   - A. crooked streets
   - B. parks
   - C. art galleries
   - D. churches
   - E. broad avenues

6. The group formed the SEMICIRCLE quickly. 6.____
   - A. half-circle
   - B. double circle
   - C. complete circle
   - D. uneven
   - E. very small circle

7. The machine that he designed was PORTABLE. 7.____
   - A. business-like
   - B. practical
   - C. of foreign manufacture
   - D. easily transported
   - E. difficult to use

8. The food supply DWINDLED during the winter. 8.____
   - A. spoiled
   - B. became less
   - C. froze
   - D. was wasted
   - E. was rationed

9. The vase was one of the PERMANENT exhibits at the museum. 9.____
   - A. historical
   - B. lasting
   - C. popular
   - D. artistic
   - E. well-planned

10. We could not understand why he left so ABRUPTLY. 10.____
    - A. suddenly
    - B. soon
    - C. absent-mindedly
    - D. mysteriously
    - E. noisily

KEY (CORRECT ANSWERS)

1. A
2. C
3. E
4. A
5. E
6. A
7. D
8. B
9. B
10. A

WORD MEANING
EXAMINATION SECTION
TEST 1

DIRECTIONS: For the following questions, select the word or group of words lettered A, B, C, D, or E that means MOST NEARLY the same as the word in capital letters. *PRINT THE LETTER OF THE CORRECT ANSWER IN THE SPACE AT THE RIGHT.*

1. The directors plan to EXPAND the factory. 1.____
   A. shut down B. remodel C. enlarge D. erect E. occupy

2. The CAPTIVE pleaded for mercy. 2.____
   A. savage B. spy C. jailer D. officer E. prisoner

3. The policeman CONSOLED the weeping child. 3.____
   A. found B. carried home C. scolded
   D. comforted E. played with

4. On these slopes there is very little VEGETATION. 4.____
   A. traffic B. rocky soil C. plant life
   D. moisture E. bird life

5. The pupil was criticized for his SLIPSHOD work. 5.____
   A. slow B. childish C. uncompleted
   D. careless E. incorrect

6. The names of characters in plays are usually FICTITIOUS. 6.____
   A. odd B. imaginary C. pleasant-sounding
   D. easy to remember E. well-known

7. The most interesting part of the book was the PREFACE. 7.____
   A. title page B. introduction C. table of contents
   D. cover design E. illustrations

8. The bullet PENETRATED the wall. 8.____
   A. entered into B. dented C. bounded off
   D. passed over E. weakened

9. The large mustache made the actor look VILLAINOUS. 9.____
   A. dignified B. slightly older C. very wicked
   D. untidy E. uncomfortable

10. They hoped to EXTERMINATE the insects. 10.____
    A. destroy B. collect C. classify
    D. experiment with E. drive away

11. It is my CONVICTION that you are wrong.
    A. fear   B. fault   C. firm belief   D. imagination   E. recollection

12. A good employee is always PUNCTUAL.
    A. polite   B. neat   C. thoughtful   D. prompt   E. truthful

13. The actor played a JUVENILE role.
    A. lovesick   B. humorous   C. criminal   D. modern   E. youthful

14. In business letters we state our business CONCISELY.
    A. accurately   B. fully   C. briefly   D. politely   E. officially

15. We found that the goods on sale were of INFERIOR quality.
    A. second-rate   B. excellent   C. lasting
    D. noticeable   E. surprising

KEY (CORRECT ANSWERS)

1. C
2. E
3. D
4. C
5. D

6. B
7. B
8. A
9. C
10. A

11. C
12. D
13. E
14. C
15. A

TEST 2

DIRECTIONS: For the following questions, select the word or group of words lettered A, B, C, D, or E that means MOST NEARLY the same as the word in capital letters. *PRINT THE LETTER OF THE CORRECT ANSWER IN THE SPACE AT THE RIGHT.*

1. The sword has a KEEN edge.

    A. bright   B. sharp   C. steel   D. polished   E. rough

2. He STARTLED the boy who was trying to unlock the car.

    A. surprised   B. punished   C. chased   D. arrested   E. helped

3. FORTHCOMING events were listed on the club bulletin board.

    A. weekly   B. interesting   C. outstanding
    D. social   E. approaching

4. The lawyer's next question ASTOUNDED the witness.

    A. misled   B. amazed   C. depressed   D. pleased   E. angered

5. In his hand the hiker was carrying a large STAFF.

    A. pack   B. loaf   C. stick
    D. musical instrument   E. garment

6. We nervously awaited the doctor's VERDICT.

    A. arrival   B. call   C. approval
    D. decision   E. prescription

7. The hikers noticed several CREVICES in the rocks.

    A. plants   B. uneven spots   C. fossils
    D. water holes   E. cracks

8. Such training helps to make a boy SELF-SUFFICIENT.

    A. clever   B. healthy   C. conceited
    D. independent   E. uncomfortable

9. The door was left AJAR.

    A. slightly opened   B. unhinged   C. unguarded
    D. unlocked   E. completely blocked

10. They talked about INSIGNIFICANT matters.

    A. unimportant   B. thrilling   C. puzzling
    D. unpleasant   E. secret

11. The child was given a good mark for DEPORTMENT.

    A. intelligence B. attendance C. health D. behavior E. neatness

12. Because of PRIOR engagements, she refused the invitation.

    A. personal B. more urgent C. more attractive
    D. future   E. earlier

13. The delegates will CONVENE at noon.

    A. dine B. vote C. debate D. assemble E. agree

14. Modern methods bring more REVENUE to the farmer.

    A. taxes B. income C. produce D. leisure E. acreage

15. The machine has MANUAL controls.

    A. self-acting B. double C. hand-operated
    D. simple   E. handmade

KEY (CORRECT ANSWERS)

1. B   6. D
2. A   7. E
3. E   8. D
4. B   9. A
5. C   10. A

11. D
12. E
13. D
14. B
15. C

TEST 3

DIRECTIONS: For the following questions, select the word or group of words lettered A, B, C, D, or E that means MOST NEARLY the same as the word in capital letters. *PRINT THE LETTER OF THE CORRECT ANSWER IN THE SPACE AT THE RIGHT.*

1. Grandfather ACQUIRED ten acres of pasture land.

    A. obtained   B. plowed   C. sold   D. leased   E. desired

2. A feeling of EXHAUSTION came over the players during the game.

    A. fear
    D. unsteadiness
    B. extreme tiredness
    E. complete happiness
    C. overconfidence

3. We pitied the child in the GRIMY clothes.

    A. ill-fitting
    D. dirty
    B. secondhand
    E. ragged
    C. poorly made

4. The mechanic's calculations were APPROXIMATE.

    A. nearly exact
    D. worthless
    B. remarkable
    E. mathematically correct
    C. hastily made

5. A COMPETENT young woman was given the position.

    A. busy
    D. friendly
    B. pretty
    E. good-natured
    C. capable

6. We had BARELY finished by six o'clock.

    A. easily
    D. more or less
    B. only just
    E. unexpectedly
    C. partly

7. His second offense was more GRIEVOUS than his first. GRIEVOUS means *most nearly*

    A. serious   B. stupid   C. deliberate   D. excusable   E. peculiar

8. All air traffic was SUSPENDED during the emergency.

    A. turned back
    D. relieved
    B. speeded up
    E. repaired
    C. stopped

9. The antics of the monkeys DIVERTED the children.

    A. upset   B. amused   C. surprised   D. disgusted   E. frightened

10. The man SURVIVED his three sisters.

    A. loved   B. envied   C. outlived   D. destroyed   E. excelled

11. Franklin was a man of EXCEPTIONAL ability.

    A. well-trained   B. active   C. mechanical
    D. self-educated   E. unusual

12. Their aim seems to be to THWART our plans.

    A. simplify   B. direct   C. rely on
    D. block   E. keep up with

13. He heard the warning cry of another PEDESTRIAN.

    A. agent   B. walker   C. passenger
    D. workingman   E. traffic officer

14. They boasted about the SUPERIORITY of their product.

    A. beauty   B. abundance   C. excellence
    D. popularity   E. permanence

15. We considered their point of view ABSURD.

    A. disgusting   B. old-fashioned   C. insincere
    D. reasonable   E. foolish

KEY (CORRECT ANSWERS)

1. A   6. B
2. B   7. A
3. D   8. C
4. A   9. B
5. C   10. C

11. E
12. D
13. B
14. C
15. E

TEST 4

DIRECTIONS: For the following questions, select the word or group of words lettered A, B, C, D, or E that means MOST NEARLY the same as the word in capital letters. *PRINT THE LETTER OF THE CORRECT ANSWER IN THE SPACE AT THE RIGHT.*

1. Our neighbor PURCHASED his home last year. 1.____
   A. bought   B. rented   C. painted   D. remodeled   E. built

2. The only sound was the STEADY ticking of the clock. 2.____
   A. noisy   B. rapid   C. regular   D. cheerful   E. tiresome

3. The desks in our room are STATIONARY. 3.____
   A. heavy   B. not movable   C. metal
   D. easily adjustable   E. standard

4. Before signing the papers, Mr. Edmond consulted his ATTORNEY. 4.____
   A. banker   B. clerk   C. lawyer   D. secretary   E. employer

5. We IMITATE those whom we admire. 5.____
   A. protect   B. attract   C. study   D. copy   E. appreciate

6. They reached the SUMMIT of the mountain by noon. 6.____
   A. base   B. wooded area   C. side
   D. face   E. top

7. The motorist HEEDED the signals. 7.____
   A. worried about   B. passed by   C. took notice of
   D. laughed at   E. disagreed with

8. The SEVERITY of their criticism upset us. 8.____
   A. purpose   B. harshness   C. method
   D. suddenness   E. unfairness

9. We made a very LEISURELY trip to California. 9.____
   A. roundabout   B. unhurried   C. unforgettable
   D. tiresome   E. speedy

10. The little girl shook her head VIGOROUSLY. 10.____
    A. sadly   B. hopefully   C. sleepily
    D. thoughtfully E. energetically

KEYS (CORRECT ANSWERS)

1. A
2. C
3. B
4. C
5. D

6. E
7. C
8. B
9. B
10. E

WORD MEANING

EXAMINATION SECTION
TEST 1

DIRECTIONS: For the following questions, select the word or group of words lettered A, B, C, D, or E that means MOST NEARLY the same as the word in capital letters. *PRINT THE LETTER OF THE CORRECT ANSWER IN THE SPACE AT THE RIGHT.*

1. PERHAPS you misunderstood his instructions. PERHAPS means *most nearly* 1.____
   A. at least   B. happily   C. maybe   D. of course   E. surely

2. Do you think the exhibit MERITS an award? MERITS means *most nearly* 2.____
   A. deserves   B. gets   C. lacks   D. requires   E. wins

3. It was a very UNUSUAL day for April. UNUSUAL means *most nearly* 3.____
   A. cold   B. delightful   C. good   D. ordinary   E. rare

4. A single FRAGRANT rose decorated his desk. FRAGRANT means *most nearly* 4.____
   A. late-blooming   B. rambling   C. sweet-smelling
   D. wilted   E. yellow

5. The GLITTERING bead attracted the crow. GLITTERING means *most nearly* 5.____
   A. bouncing   B. colored   C. gleaming   D. pretty   E. rolling

6. Jack did NOTICE the attractive child. NOTICE means *most nearly* 6.____
   A. believe   B. observe   C. overlook   D. speak to   E. write to

7. We are too fond of the ADVANTAGES of civilization. ADVANTAGES means *most nearly* 7.____
   A. benefits   B. changes   C. classes   D. powers   E. results

8. Accidents in the home may cause INJURY. INJURY means *most nearly* 8.____
   A. danger   B. death   C. delay   D. grief   E. harm

9. The Spanish explorers found great TREASURES for their king. TREASURES means *most nearly* 9.____
   A. banks   B. chests   C. islands   D. riches   E. values

10. They prepared a great BANQUET for the returning general. BANQUET means *most nearly* 10.____
    A. ball   B. feast   C. gift   D. hall   E. surprise

11. We must learn to be TOLERANT of people different from ourselves. TOLERANT means *most nearly* 11.____
    A. afraid   B. aware   C. careful   D. suspicious
    E. understanding

12. His AMBITION caused him to go to night school. AMBITION means *most nearly*   12.____
    A. desire to succeed B. fortune C. hope of freedom
    D. ignorance E. pride

13. The frightened child ran to EMBRACE her mother. EMBRACE means *most nearly*   13.____
    A. call B. escape C. hug D. scold E. watch

14. ACTUALLY he did not know the man. ACTUALLY means *most nearly*   14.____
    A. now B. often C. really D. suddenly E. then

15. The hike up Mount Marcy was STRENUOUS. STRENUOUS means *most nearly*   15.____
    A. disappointing B. dull C. pleasant
    D. scenic E. vigorous

KEY (CORRECT ANSWERS)

1. C   6. B
2. A   7. A
3. E   8. E
4. C   9. D
5. C   10. B

11. E
12. A
13. C
14. C
15. E

TEST 2

DIRECTIONS: For the following questions, select the word or group of words lettered A, B, C, D, or E that means MOST NEARLY the same as the word in capital letters. *PRINT THE LETTER OF THE CORRECT ANSWER IN THE SPACE AT THE RIGHT.*

1. The traveler carried SUFFICIENT money for the trip. SUFFICIENT means *most nearly* 1._____

    A. counterfeit   B. enough   C. less
    D. too little   E. too much

2. He walked HASTILY to the counter. HASTILY means *most nearly* 2._____

    A. angrily   B. often   C. quickly   D. seldom   E. slowly

3. I shall CONCEAL the letter in the tree. CONCEAL means *most nearly* 3._____

    A. catch   B. find   C. hide   D. steal   E. throw

4. He prefers to DWELL in the country. DWELL means *most nearly* 4._____

    A. build   B. picnic   C. rent   D. live   E. continue

5. There is no CERTAIN way of locating their treasure. CERTAIN means *most nearly* 5._____

    A. better   B. easy   C. familiar   D. private   E. sure

6. In FORMER times life was more simple. FORMER means *most nearly* 6._____

    A. better   B. later   C. earlier   D. happier   E. calmer

7. The immigrant's arrival marked the COMMENCEMENT of a new life. COMMENCEMENT means *most nearly* 7._____

    A. beginning   B. choosing   C. finishing   D. seeking   E. settling

8. The war brought the people much MISERY. MISERY means *most nearly* 8._____

    A. distress   B. distrust   C. toil   D. hatred   E. money

9. The teacher was EXTREMELY pleased with her students. EXTREMELY means *most nearly* 9._____

    A. seldom   B. often   C. sometimes   D. frequently   E. very

10. The trapper INDICATED the streams where fishing was best. INDICATED means *most nearly* 10._____

    A. described   B. kept secret   C. pointed out
    D. retraced   E. walked along

11. The odd results of the experiment PERPLEXED the scientists. PERPLEXED means *most nearly* 11._____

    A. decided   B. disgusted   C. helped   D. puzzled   E. surprised

12. The hostess greeted the guest CORDIALLY. CORDIALLY means *most nearly*

    A. unpleasantly   B. coldly   C. crudely   D. heartily
    E. sentimentally

13. Do not CONFUSE the audience when you speak. CONFUSE means *most nearly*

    A. tire   B. bewilder   C. consider   D. criticize   E. forget

14. The HOSTILE attitude of my neighbor frightened me. HOSTILE means *most nearly*

    A. doubtful   B. friendly   C. indifferent
    D. suspicious   E. unfriendly

15. How long do you think you can ENDURE these conditions? ENDURE means *most nearly*

    A. await   B. bear   C. demand   D. escape   E. obey

KEY (CORRECT ANSWERS)

1. B
2. C
3. C
4. D
5. E
6. C
7. A
8. A
9. E
10. C
11. D
12. D
13. B
14. E
15. B

TEST 3

DIRECTIONS: For the following questions, select the word or group of words lettered A, B, C, D, or E that means MOST NEARLY the same as the word in capital letters. *PRINT THE LETTER OF THE CORRECT ANSWER IN THE SPACE AT THE RIGHT.*

1. The office manager was given considerable LATITUDE insetting up the procedures for the new unit. LATITUDE means *most nearly*   1._____

    A. advice and encouragement
    B. assistance and cooperation
    C. cause for annoyance
    D. freedom from restriction
    E. freedom from fear

2. He said that this was an EXPEDIENT method of performing the job. EXPEDIENT means *most nearly*   2._____

    A. inconvenient and ineffective
    B. effective but expensive
    C. practical and efficient
    D. convenient but time consuming
    E. forceful but necessary

3. The men refused to give up their PREROGATIVES without a struggle. PREROGATIVES means *most nearly*   3._____

    A. ideals   B. demands   C. rights   D. advantages   E. exemptions

4. Shakespeare was a PROLIFIC writer. PROLIFIC means *most nearly*   4._____

    A. productive   B. popular   C. richly talented
    D. forward-looking   E. enigmatic

5. His electric lines are in close PROXIMITY with mine. PROXIMITY means *most nearly*   5._____

    A. nearness
    B. appropriateness
    C. identity
    D. necessity
    E. prolixity

6. The situation presented an unanticipated DILEMMA to the supervisor. DILEMMA means *most nearly*   6._____

    A. procedure
    B. solution
    C. opportunity
    D. assignment
    E. predicament

7. The population of a city is generally more HETEROGENEOUS than that of a rural community. HETEROGENEOUS means *most nearly*   7._____

    A. mixed   B. competent   C. unhealthy   D. prosperous   E. unique

8. His mother is a FRUGAL person. FRUGAL means *most nearly*   8._____

    A. discontented
    B. cheerful
    C. untruthful
    D. thrifty
    E. profound

9. Their interests were INIMICAL to the objectives of the organization. INIMICAL means *most nearly*

    A. opposed   B. agreeable   C. related   D. essential   E. unlike

10. He is an ECCENTRIC old man. ECCENTRIC means *most nearly*

    A. wealthy   B. self-centered
    C. envious   D. peculiar
    E. extravagant

11. The caller's manner was FURTIVE. FURTIVE means *most nearly*

    A. careless   B. sly   C. forceful   D. aloof   E. frivolous

12. The clerk CORROBORATED the stenographer's report. CORROBORATED means *most nearly*

    A. contradicted   B. confirmed
    C. summarized   D. corrected
    E. questioned

13. The manager dictated a TERSE letter. TERSE means *most nearly*

    A. angry   B. coherent   C. brief   D. lengthy   E. tearful

14. The EMINENT visitor drew all eyes. EMINENT means *most nearly*

    A. menacing   B. uninvited   C. awkward   D. tall   E. notable

15. Her quiet tone MITIGATED his anxiety. MITIGATED means *most nearly*

    A. intensified   B. alleviated   C. ridiculed   D. provoked   E. belied

---

KEY (CORRECT ANSWERS)

1. D   6. E
2. C   7. A
3. C   8. D
4. A   9. A
5. A   10. D

11. B
12. B
13. C
14. E
15. B

TEST 4

DIRECTIONS: For the following questions, select the word or group of words lettered A, B, C, D, or E that means MOST NEARLY the same as the word in capital letters. *PRINT THE LETTER OF THE CORRECT ANSWER IN THE SPACE AT THE RIGHT.*

1. The extinguisher must be INVERTED before it will operate. INVERTED means *most nearly*

   A. turned over B. completely filled C. lightly shaken
   D. unhooked E. opened

   1.____

2. Sprinkler systems in buildings can RETARD the spread of fires. RETARD means *most nearly*

   A. quench B. outline C. slow D. reveal E. aggravate

   2.____

3. Although there was widespread criticism, the director refused to CURTAIL the program. CURTAIL means *most nearly*

   A. change B. discuss C. shorten D. expand E. enforce

   3.____

4. Argon is an INERT gas. INERT means *most nearly*

   A. unstable B. uncommon C. volatile D. inferior E. inactive

   4.____

5. The firemen turned their hoses on the shed and the main building SIMULTANEOUSLY. SIMULTANEOUSLY means *most nearly*

   A. in turn B. without hesitation C. with great haste
   D. as needed E. at the same time

   5.____

6. The officer was REBUKED for his failure to act promptly. REBUKED means *most nearly*

   A. demoted B. reprimanded
   C. discharged D. reassigned
   E. suspended

   6.____

7. Parkways in the city may be used to FACILITATE responses to alarms. FACILITATE means *most nearly*

   A. reduce B. alter C. complete D. ease E. control

   7.____

8. Fire extinguishers are most effective when the fire is INCIPIENT. INCIPIENT means *most nearly*

   A. accessible B. beginning C. red hot D. confined E. smoky

   8.____

9. It is important to CONVEY TO new members the fundamental methods of firefighting. CONVEY TO means *most nearly*

   A. inquire of B. prove for C. confirm for
   D. suggest to E. impart to

   9.____

10. The explosion was a GRAPHIC illustration of the effects of neglect and carelessness. GRAPHIC means *most nearly*

    A. terrible B. poor C. typical D. unique E. vivid

    10.____

11. The fireman was ASSIDUOUS in all things relating to his duties. ASSIDUOUS means most nearly

    A. aggressive   B. careless   C. persistent   D. cautious   E. dogmatic

12. A fireman must be ADEPT to be successful at his work. ADEPT means most nearly

    A. ambitious   B. strong   C. agile   D. alert   E. skillful

13. Officers shall see that parts are issued in CONSECUTIVE order. CONSECUTIVE means most nearly

    A. objective   B. random   C. conducive   D. effective   E. successive

14. Practically every municipality has fire ORDINANCES. ORDINANCES means most nearly

    A. drills   B. stations   C. engines   D. laws   E. problems

15. When the smoke cleared away, the firemen's task was ALLEVIATED. ALLEVIATED means most nearly

    A. lessened   B. visible   C. appreciated
    D. safer   E. accomplished

KEY (CORRECT ANSWERS)

1. A
2. C
3. C
4. E
5. E
6. B
7. D
8. B
9. E
10. E
11. C
12. E
13. E
14. D
15. A

VOCABULARY
SAME (SYNONYMS)
TEST 1

DIRECTIONS: Each question in this part consists of a word in capital letters, followed by four words lettered A, B, C, D. Choose the letter of the word that is MOST NEARLY the same in meaning to the word in capital letters. *PRINT THE LETTER OF THE CORRECT ANSWER IN THE SPACE AT THE RIGHT.*

1. EXTANT
   - A. length
   - B. space
   - C. in existence
   - D. utterly destroyed

2. EXUDE
   - A. discharge
   - B. cut out
   - C. drive away
   - D. leave hastily

3. FEIGN
   - A. temporize
   - B. oscillate
   - C. be eager
   - D. simulate

4. FELICITY
   - A. savagery
   - B. duplicity
   - C. misfortune
   - D. happiness

5. FILCH
   - A. shrink
   - B. pilfer
   - C. cut into strips
   - D. besmirch

6. GARRULITY
   - A. talkativeness
   - B. silence
   - C. old age
   - D. foolishness

7. HAGGLE
   - A. purchase
   - B. fish
   - C. become gaunt
   - D. dispute

8. HAWSER
   - A. soldier
   - B. rope
   - C. sail
   - D. anchor

9. INTERMENT
   - A. burial
   - B. shroud
   - C. funeral
   - D. sepulchre

10. INUNDATE
    - A. irrigate
    - B. empty
    - C. flood
    - D. ruin

11. INVEIGLE
    - A. attack
    - B. lure
    - C. suspect
    - D. blind

69

2 (#1)

12. JOSTLE

   A. trip   B. elbow   C. bully   D. rob

13. LACONIC

   A. indifferent   B. talkative
   C. concise   D. distinct

14. LATENT

   A. apparent   B. meaningful
   C. not punctual   D. hidden

15. MALIGN

   A. slander   B. pretend illness
   C. pity   D. wear away

16. MODICUM

   A. measure   B. average
   C. small portion   D. praise

17. MYRIAD

   A. constellation   B. large number
   C. water nymph   D. warrior

18. OBDURATE

   A. penetrating   B. unyielding
   C. lasting a long time   D. objecting

19. ONEROUS

   A. laudatory   B. burdensome
   C. detailed   D. qualitative

20. OSTRACIZE

   A. cut   B. snub   C. burn   D. banish

21. PARAGON

   A. geometric figure   B. beauty
   C. model   D. virtue

22. PEER

   A. dock   B. nobleman   C. citizen   D. rank

23. PENURIOUS

   A. irritable   B. lavish
   C. poor   D. dangerous

24. PERENNIAL

   A. enduring   B. yearly
   C. lasting only a year D. every two years

3 (#1)

25. PERNICIOUS   25._____
    A. fussy   B. diseased   C. hurtful   D. lying

26. PHILOLOGY   26._____
    A. study of love   B. wisdom
    C. grammar   D. linguistic science

27. POSTULATE   27._____
    A. afterthought   B. hypothesis
    C. blister   D. riding horseback

28. POTENT   28._____
    A. mighty   B. poisonous
    C. pleasant   D. uncompromising

29. PROGNOSIS   29._____
    A. analysis   B. recognition of symptoms
    C. forecast   D. testing results

30. PROPITIATE   30._____
    A. attract   B. advertise   C. appease   D. propose

31. PUNCTILIOUS   31._____
    A. prompt   B. full of punctuation
    C. full of perforation   D. scrupulous

32. QUANDARY   32._____
    A. predicament   B. amount
    C. contrariness   D. quarrel

33. RANKLE   33._____
    A. produce a soothing effect
    B. fester
    C. keep repeating
    D. produce convolutions

34. REDRESS   34._____
    A. clothe   B. send   C. remedy   D. wrong

35. SAGACIOUS   35._____
    A. pertaining to a gland   B. wise
    C. pertaining to a song   D. mythical

36. SANGUINARY   36._____
    A. murderous   B. hopeful   C. decisive   D. pugnacious

37. SAVOR   37._____
    A. help   B. cook   C. approve   D. relish

38. SCION

    A. black sheep B. renegade
    C. scholar   D. heir

39. SHIBBOLETH

    A. war cry   B. secret
    C. watchword   D. holy word

40. SIDLE

    A. fizz   B. slink
    C. move sidewise D. sit

41. SLEAZY

    A. easy   B. flimsy
    C. made of wool D. coarse

42. SPASMODIC

    A. continuous B. intermittent
    C. feverish   D. gradual

43. SPECIOUS

    A. belonging to a variety B. financial
    C. easily observed   D. plausible

44. SULLY

    A. condemn   B. assail   C. dirty   D. sour

45. SWAB

    A. mop   B. exchange   C. saturate   D. medicate

46. SYLPH

    A. imaginary being B. emblem
    C. tiny beetle   D. forest

47. TALISMAN

    A. charm   B. juror   C. perjurer   D. magician

48. TOXIC

    A. sleepy   B. pertaining to liquor
    C. drugged D. pertaining to poison

49. TURPITUDE

    A. sluggishness B. dishonesty
    C. depravity   D. confusion

50. UPBRAID

    A. weave   B. reproach   C. twist   D. decorate

KEY (CORRECT ANSWERS)

1. C	11. B	21. C	31. D	41. B
2. A	12. B	22. B	32. A	42. B
3. D	13. C	23. C	33. B	43. D
4. D	14. D	24. A	34. C	44. C
5. B	15. A	25. C	35. B	45. A
6. A	16. C	26. D	36. A	46. A
7. D	17. B	27. B	37. D	47. A
8. B	18. B	28. A	38. D	48. D
9. A	19. B	29. C	39. C	49. C
10. C	20. D	30. C	40. C	50. B

TEST 2

DIRECTIONS: Each question in this part consists of a word in capital letters, followed by four words lettered A, B, C, D. Choose the letter of the word that is MOST NEARLY the same in meaning to the word in capital letters. *PRINT THE LETTER OF THE CORRECT ANSWER IN THE SPACE AT THE RIGHT.*

1. NOISOME
   - A. disgusting
   - B. loud
   - C. irritating
   - D. rambunctious

   1.____

2. NOSTALGIC
   - A. bouquet
   - B. disgust
   - C. seasick
   - D. homesick

   2.____

3. OFFICIOUS
   - A. useful
   - B. meddlesome
   - C. generous
   - D. urbane

   3.____

4. OMNIPOTENT
   - A. inform
   - B. impressive
   - C. ubiquitous
   - D. almighty

   4.____

5. OROTUND
   - A. pompous
   - B. underground
   - C. impecunious
   - D. obese

   5.____

6. OSTENTATIOUS
   - A. pretentious
   - B. wonderful
   - C. of great extent
   - D. inconspicuous

   6.____

7. PAROXYSM
   - A. paralysis
   - B. comedy
   - C. mental disorder
   - D. violent outburst

   7.____

8. PARRY
   - A. return
   - B. delay
   - C. discuss
   - D. ward off

   8.____

9. PENCHANT
   - A. Australian insect
   - B. symbol of victory
   - C. ornamental neck-piece
   - D. a particular inclination

   9.____

10. PERSIFLAGE
    - A. verbosity
    - B. banter
    - C. deception
    - D. intrigue

    10.____

11. PERTINENT
    - A. bold
    - B. respectful
    - C. relevant
    - D. humble

    11.____

74

2 (#2)

12. PLEBISCITE 12.____
    A. type of stone B. vulgarity
    C. peasantry D. popular vote

13. PLENARY 13.____
    A. flexible B. pleasing
    C. superfluous D. complete

14. PRECURSOR 14.____
    A. heathen B. blasphemer
    C. forerunner D. calumniator

15. PREDATORY 15.____
    A. inherited B. precocious
    C. plundering D. divine

16. PROPITIOUS 16.____
    A. near B. hasty C. ominous D. favorable

17. QUERULOUS 17.____
    A. complaining B. inquisitive
    C. argumentative D. evasive

18. RAUCOUS 18.____
    A. disagreeably harsh B. native
    C. original D. freshly selected

19. RECLUSE 19.____
    A. hypocrite B. hermit
    C. gourmand D. epicure

20. RECONDITE 20.____
    A. carefully surveyed B. exhaustive
    C. profound D. of high character

21. RECUMBENT 21.____
    A. heavy B. obligatory
    C. reclining D. superfluous

22. REDUNDANT 22.____
    A. resounding B. excessive
    C. renowned D. returning

23. RENEGADE 23.____
    A. murderer B. deserter C. rebel D. hypocrite

24. REPLETE 24.____

3 (#2)

    A. conducive   B. impetuous
    C. plentiful   D. scarce

25. RESCIND
    A. to admit error
    B. to retreat from a position
    C. to apologize and make amends
    D. to repeal or abrogate

25.____

26. RIBALD
    A. hairless   B. stern
    C. coarsely jocular   D. impressionable

26.____

27. RIFE
    A. mature   B. prevalent
    C. auspicious   D. ready

27.____

28. SANGUINE
    A. hopeful   B. malicious
    C. inferior   D. without cause

28.____

29. SCHISM
    A. division   B. sheets of rock
    C. descendant   D. saber

29.____

30. SLAKE
    A. endure   B. quench   C. strike   D. criticize

30.____

31. SLOTH
    A. gluttony   B. inebriety
    C. indolence   D. mire

31.____

32. SPECIOUS
    A. plausible   B. coins   C. culled   D. specific

32.____

33. SPORADIC
    A. exotic   B. occasional
    C. unimportant   D. wandering

33.____

34. SPURIOUS
    A. wretched   B. unfortunate
    C. false   D. illogical

34.____

35. SUBVERSIVE
    A. controversial   B. destructive
    C. un-American   D. changeable

35.____

36. SUPINE

36.____

A. suppliant   B. prostrate
C. conquered   D. refined

37. SURFEIT   37.____

    A. delegate   B. confiscate
    C. corroborate   D. satiate

38. SYCOPHANT   38.____

    A. follower   B. small elephant
    C. warrior   D. flatterer

39. TACITURN   39.____

    A. reticent   B. loquacious
    C. saturnine   D. sullen

40. TANTAMOUNT   40.____

    A. equal   B. mountebank
    C. repetitious   D. unequal parts

41. TENET   41.____

    A. decimal   B. grasp   C. joint   D. doctrine

42. TRUCULENT   42.____

    A. toilsome   B. fierce   C. dull   D. mild

43. TUMESCENT   43.____

    A. fragrant   B. swelling
    C. exemplary   D. resentful

44. UBIQUITOUS   44.____

    A. courteous   B. deceased
    C. ever-present   D. silenced

45. VACILLATE   45.____

    A. obscure   B. waver   C. differ   D. prevent

46. VIRULENT   46.____

    A. manly   B. verdant C. injurious D. widespread

47. WARY   47.____

    A. distorted   B. bellicose
    C. vigilant   D. exhausted

48. WAYWARD   48.____

    A. exhausted   B. underage
    C. on the beaten track   D. perverse

49. WRAITH

    A. avenger
    C. dispute
    B. specter
    D. floral tribute

50. ZANY

    A. magician
    C. clown
    B. fortune-teller
    D. hypnotist

KEY (CORRECT ANSWERS)

1. A	11. C	21. C	31. C	41. D
2. D	12. D	22. B	32. A	42. B
3. B	13. D	23. B	33. B	43. B
4. D	14. C	24. C	34. C	44. C
5. A	15. C	25. D	35. B	45. B
6. A	16. D	26. C	36. B	46. C
7. D	17. A	27. B	37. D	47. C
8. D	18. A	28. A	38. D	48. D
9. D	19. B	29. A	39. A	49. B
10. B	20. C	30. B	40. A	50. C

TEST 3

DIRECTIONS: Each question in this part consists of a word in capital letters, followed by four words lettered A, B, C, D. Choose the letter of the word that is MOST NEARLY the same in meaning to the word in capital letters. *PRINT THE LETTER OF THE CORRECT ANSWER IN THE SPACE AT THE RIGHT.*

1. MARAUDER
   A. prize-fighter   B. fish
   C. seafaring man   D. plunderer

   1.___

2. MARROW
   A. muscle   B. tendon   C. pith   D. gristle

   2.___

3. MAUL
   A. handle roughly   B. stroke lovingly
   C. speak gruffly   D. walk heavily

   3.___

4. METICULOUS
   A. picayune   B. overscrupulous
   C. plodding   D. brilliant

   4.___

5. METTLE
   A. irritation   B. medallion
   C. obstinacy   D. courage

   5.___

6. MIEN
   A. character   B. appearance
   C. disposition   D. reputation

   6.___

7. MIRAGE
   A. optical phenomenon   B. acute visibility
   C. clear perception   D. divine apparition

   7.___

8. MISSILE
   A. letter   B. prayer book
   C. messenger   D. weapon

   8.___

9. MONSOON
   A. gentlemen   B. wind
   C. bird   D. wild animal

   9.___

10. MORASS
    A. beg   B. ditch   C. oak   D. treacle

    10.___

11. NECTAR
    A. condiment   B. juicy fruit
    C. sweet drink   D. bitter herb

    11.___

12. NEFARIOUS
    A. sea-going B. sinful C. doubtful D. tough

13. NOMAD
    A. hermit B. caveman C. wanderer D. yokel

14. NOSEGAY
    A. homesickness B. bouquet
    C. compliment D. handkerchief

15. NUPTIAL
    A. conjugal B. barbaric
    C. hymnal D. celibate

16. OBLOQUY
    A. disgrace B. forgetfulness
    C. fame D. popularity

17. OBSEQUIES
    A. burial service B. shrouds
    C. cringing actions D. atonement for sins

18. ODIOUS
    A. pungent B. lyrical C. quaint D. repugnant

19. OSCILLATE
    A. vibrate B. kiss
    C. elevate D. set fractures

20. OSTENSIBLE
    A. gaudy B. stubborn C. apparent D. elastic

21. PARCH
    A. spank B. scorch C. rest D. skin

22. PARRICIDE
    A. regicide B. disease
    C. parental murder D. at the side of

23. PERVADE
    A. mislead B. endure C. permeate D. deter

24. PETULANT
    A. cross B. worried C. pleading D. pampered

25. PIQUE
    A. sly look B. sauciness
    C. selection D. resentment

26. PORTENT
    A. corpulent   B. omen   C. carrier   D. gate

27. PROFLIGATE
    A. lavish   B. fruitful   C. immoral   D. beneficial

28. QUALM
    A. scruple   B. bird   C. serenity   D. repose

29. RECALCITRANT
    A. receptive   B. resistant   C. adaptable   D. profane

30. RECIDIVIST
    A. dramatist   B. reciter
    C. confirmed criminal   D. pensioner

31. RECREANT
    A. accusing   B. refreshing
    C. amusing   D. cowardly

32. SARDONIC
    A. doomed   B. derisive   C. electronic   D. astral

33. SCOURGE
    A. purge   B. vulgarity
    C. vitamin deficiency   D. whip

34. SCULLION
    A. unrefined metal   B. servant
    C. vegetable   D. brain injury

35. SEDIMENT
    A. inactivity   B. emotion
    C. treason   D. dregs

36. SIMULATE
    A. concur   B. transform   C. imitate   D. encourage

37. SINEW
    A. tendon   B. tough skin
    C. curve   D. evil deed

38. SINISTER
    A. skeptical   B. inconsiderate
    C. awkward   D. malevolent

39. SOJOURN
    A. meander   B. assemble   C. stay   D. dismiss

40. SPAWN
    A. cast aside   B. deposit eggs
    C. tend hay   D. swim upstream

41. SQUALID
    A. stocky   B. bawling   C. filthy   D. stormy

42. STIGMA
    A. blemish   B. eye defect
    C. inertia   D. ornament

43. SUCCULENT
    A. gullible   B. unweaned   C. helpful   D. juicy

44. SYMMETRICAL
    A. concave   B. changeable
    C. approximate   D. well-balanced

45. SYNCHRONOUS
    A. simultaneous   B. accented
    C. disjointed   D. melodious

46. TEMPORIZE
    A. soothe   B. infuriate
    C. procrastinate   D. inflame

47. TRAVESTY
    A. expedition   B. cross-beam
    C. burlesque   D. needle

48. TRELLIS
    A. lattice   B. chromatic scale
    C. lever   D. fishing boat

49. TROWEL
    A. garden tool   B. fishing reel
    C. coping saw   D. wheelbarrow

50. VIADUCT
    A. pipe   B. levee
    C. bridge   D. railroad bed

KEY (CORRECT ANSWERS)

1. D	11. C	21. B	31. D	41. C
2. C	12. B	22. C	32. B	42. A
3. A	13. C	23. C	33. D	43. D
4. B	14. B	24. A	34. B	44. D
5. D	15. A	25. D	35. D	45. A
6. B	16. A	26. B	36. C	46. C
7. A	17. A	27. C	37. A	47. C
8. D	18. D	28. A	38. D	48. A
9. B	19. A	29. B	39. C	49. A
10. A	20. C	30. C	40. B	50. C

TEST 4

DIRECTIONS: Each question in this part consists of a word in capital letters, followed by four words lettered A, B, C, D. Choose the letter of the word that is MOST NEARLY the same in meaning to the word in capital letters. *PRINT THE LETTER OF THE CORRECT ANSWER IN THE SPACE AT THE RIGHT.*

1. INTERSTICES 1.____
   A. scare B. decrees C. spaces D. nets

2. ITINERANT 2.____
   A. begging B. wandering C. erring D. metallic

3. JETTISON 3.____
   A. garrison B. throw overboard
   C. fasten down D. loosen

4. LACONIC 4.____
   A. watery B. narrow C. geometric D. terse

5. LAISSEZ-FAIRE 5.____
   A. each to his own taste
   B. evil to him who evil thinks
   C. equal justice
   D. non-interference

6. LURID 6.____
   A. black and blue B. pale
   C. dry D. destructive

7. MALINGER 7.____
   A. cheat B. delay
   C. suffer D. feign illness

8. MELANCHOLY 8.____
   A. lamentable B. garrulous
   C. fulsome D. dour

9. MORBID 9.____
   A. angry B. dying
   C. diseased D. irritated

10. MORDANT 10.____
    A. blended B. ridiculing
    C. shy D. biting

11. MORES 11.____
    A. procrastination B. ethics
    C. legends D. customs

12. NEBULOUS   12.____

    A. nascent   B. idealistic
    C. bubbling   D. indefinite

13. OBSECRATE   13.____

    A. conceal   B. defile   C. entreat   D. sanctify

14. OBTUSE   14.____

    A. stupid   B. difficult   C. unpopular   D. recondite

15. OPULENT   15.____

    A. affluent   B. hopeful
    C. urgent   D. comfortable

16. PALLIATE   16.____

    A. carry   B. mitigate   C. crush   D. bargain

17. PANDEMIC   17.____

    A. communal   B. local
    C. universal   D. all-knowing

18. PARIAH   18.____

    A. elder   B. outcast
    C. church district   D. Hebrew unit of measure

19. PERFUNCTORY   19.____

    A. negligent   B. meaningful
    C. courteous   D. deliberate

20. PIEBALD   20.____

    A. bright   B. animal   C. mottled   D. hairy

21. PORTENTOUS   21.____

    A. precarious   B. deadly
    C. ominous   D. poisonous

22. POTABLE   22.____

    A. soup   B. drinkable   C. wretched   D. movable

23. PRISTINE   23.____

    A. shining   B. primitive
    C. lachrymose   D. glorious

24. PROPINQUITY   24.____

    A. kinship   B. fertility
    C. eccentricity   D. stimulation

25. QUONDAM
    A. puzzled   B. former   C. flight   D. early

26. REDOLENT
    A. lazy   B. odorous   C. sleepy   D. honeyed

27. REDOUBTABLE
    A. uncertain   B. positive
    C. fortifiable   D. formidable

28. REFRACTORY
    A. glassy   B. bending   C. fusible   D. stubborn

29. REGIMEN
    A. crown   B. control
    C. group   D. military unit

30. RETICENT
    A. backward   B. rash   C. timid   D. reserved

31. RUBICUND
    A. precious   B. sparkling   C. reddish   D. rotund

32. SATURNINE
    A. planetary   B. dazzling   C. gloomy   D. stellar

33. SCINTILLA
    A. drug   B. Mexican food
    C. trace   D. bending

34. SMIRCH
    A. smile   B. tarnish   C. deride   D. singe

35. SOMATIC
    A. symptomatic   B. sleepy
    C. physical   D. worked by hand

36. SOPORIFIC
    A. pain killer   B. washing powder
    C. sweat producer   D. causing sleep

37. STACCATO
    A. disconnected   B. soft
    C. dagger   D. melodious

38. STULTIFY
    A. asphyxiate   B. ferment
    C. thicken   D. render foolish

39. SUCCINCT

    A. feeble   B. touched   C. pithy   D. verbose

40. SURREPTITIOUS

    A. sophisticated   B. savory
    C. stealthy   D. vindictive

41. TORPID

    A. of a certain color   B. lukewarm
    C. sluggish   D. swollen

42. UNCTUOUS

    A. avuncular   B. pertaining to last rites
    C. oily   D. eager

43. VALID

    A. important   B. cogent
    C. masculine   D. argumentative

44. VERDURE

    A. foliage   B. age
    C. truth   D. manly strength

45. VERNAL

    A. springlike   B. scale
    C. green   D. luxuriant

46. VIRAGO

    A. lush vegetation   B. wife
    C. green tint   D. termagant

47. VISCOUS

    A. malevolent   B. insulting
    C. sticky   D. financial

48. VITREOUS

    A. destructive   B. callous
    C. sarcastic   D. glassy

49. VOLUBLE

    A. liquid   B. talkative
    C. easy-going   D. sizable

50. ZENITH

    A. celestial sphere   B. acme
    C. nadir   D. astrology

KEY (CORRECT ANSWERS)

1. C	11. D	21. C	31. C	41. C
2. B	12. D	22. B	32. C	42. C
3. B	13. C	23. B	33. C	43. B
4. D	14. A	24. A	34. B	44. A
5. D	15. A	25. B	35. C	45. A
6. B	16. B	26. B	36. D	46. D
7. D	17. C	27. D	37. A	47. C
8. A	18. B	28. D	38. D	48. D
9. C	19. A	29. B	39. C	49. B
10. D	20. C	30. D	40. C	50. B

TEST 5

DIRECTIONS: Each question in this part consists of a word in capital letters, followed by four words lettered A, B, C, D. Choose the letter of the word that is MOST NEARLY the same in meaning to the word in capital letters. *PRINT THE LETTER OF THE CORRECT ANSWER IN THE SPACE AT THE RIGHT.*

1. FULSOME
   - A. worthy
   - B. unlimited
   - C. laudable
   - D. disgusting

2. GOURD
   - A. ornament
   - B. fruit
   - C. pipe
   - D. instrument

3. GUNWALE
   - A. part of a boat
   - B. kind of cloth
   - C. part of a basket
   - D. part of a gun

4. HYBRID
   - A. mongrel
   - B. eugenic
   - C. exaggerated
   - D. dwarfed

5. IDYLLIC
   - A. picturesque
   - B. chivalric
   - C. adoring
   - D. perfect

6. IMMINENT
   - A. direct
   - B. impending
   - C. very large
   - D. incurable

7. INTERPOLATE
   - A. make remarks
   - B. insert
   - C. criticize
   - D. edit

8. INURE
   - A. habituate
   - B. enfeeble
   - C. harm
   - D. wear out

9. JETTY
   - A. engine
   - B. pier
   - C. ebony
   - D. current

10. LARCENOUS
    - A. craven
    - B. inflamed
    - C. lewd
    - D. thieving

11. LINEAMENT
    - A. outline
    - B. medicine
    - C. face
    - D. ancestry

12. MACHIAVELLIAN
    - A. adaptable
    - B. medieval
    - C. optimistic
    - D. unscrupulous

13. MINION
    A. group B. soldier C. dependent D. flower

14. MOLLIFY
    A. humiliate B. appease C. bribe D. convince

15. MUNDANE
    A. monthly B. commercial
    C. worldly D. sinful

16. NECROMANCY
    A. neurosis B. mathematics
    C. magic D. morbidity

17. OVERWEANING
    A. conceited B. defiant
    C. outbidding D. surmounting

18. PAEAN
    A. laborer B. song C. mourning D. pouring

19. PALL
    A. vehicle B. coffin C. altar D. mantle

20. PARABLE
    A. curve B. contradiction
    C. allegory D. equal ability

21. PECULATION
    A. disease B. investment
    C. singularity D. embezzlement

22. PERDITION
    A. foolishness B. ruin
    C. rejection D. atonement

23. PERFIDY
    A. faith B. reality C. treachery D. vow

24. QUOTIDIAN
    A. ordinary B. accurate C. quaint D. archaic

25. REGALE
    A. feast B. crown C. tell D. laugh

26. RIBALD
    A. jesting B. objectionable
    C. unbridled D. coarse

27. RUDIMENTARY 27.____
    A. undeveloped   B. discourteous
    C. ill-intentioned   D. vague

28. SCALPEL 28.____
    A. tuft of hair   B. small profit
    C. small knife   D. small probe

29. SCLEROUS 29.____
    A. abusive   B. hard   C. sarcastic   D. injurious

30. SCURVY 30.____
    A. deceitful B. starving C. foul   D. mean

31. SEDULOUS 31.____
    A. ape-like   B. sitting   C. diligent   D. tiresome

32. SINUOUS 32.____
    A. strong   B. treacherous
    C. winding   D. hanging

33. SLEIGHT 33.____
    A. sledge   B. insult   C. dexterity   D. swamp

34. SNIVEL 34.____
    A. snuffle   B. swing   C. cringe   D. spit

35. STANCHION 35.____
    A. firmness B. sword   C. support   D. animal

36. SUPERCILIOUS 36.____
    A. disdainful   B. perfect
    C. nauseating   D. ill

37. TAUTOLOGY 37.____
    A. classification   B. repetitive idea
    C. science   D. theory

38. TENUOUS 38.____
    A. false   B. holding fast
    C. thin   D. simple

39. TRENCHANT 39.____
    A. hollow   B. critical C. cutting   D. saving

40. TRUSS 40.____
    A. bind   B. curse   C. sever   D. decorate

41. TYRO
    A. yodeler   B. beginner
    C. red   D. a large bow

42. ULULATE
    A. howl   B. fertilize   C. overcome   D. frolic

43. UMBRAGE
    A. burden   B. displeasure
    C. sanctimony   D. eclipse

44. UNDULATE
    A. flood   B. dress   C. decrease   D. wave

45. VERACITY
    A. fierceness   B. greed
    C. character   D. truth

46. VIRIDESCENT
    A. masculine   B. greenish
    C. resplendent   D. colorful

47. VITRIOLIC
    A. caustic   B. glassy   C. efficient   D. animated

48. VOTIVE
    A. devoted   B. selective
    C. spontaneous   D. peaceful

49. WAINSCOT
    A. wagon   B. article of clothing
    C. ceiling   D. paneling

50. WELKIN
    A. roof   B. sky   C. world   D. spring

KEY (CORRECT ANSWERS)

1. D	11. A	21. D	31. C	41. B
2. B	12. D	22. B	32. C	42. A
3. A	13. C	23. C	33. C	43. B
4. A	14. B	24. A	34. A	44. D
5. A	15. C	25. A	35. C	45. D
6. B	16. C	26. D	36. A	46. B
7. B	17. B	27. A	37. B	47. A
8. A	18. B	28. C	38. C	48. A
9. B	19. D	29. B	39. C	49. D
10. D	20. C	30. D	40. A	50. B

ANTONYMS/OPPOSITES
EXAMINATION SECTION

DIRECTIONS FOR THIS SECTION: Each question below consists of a word printed in capital letters, followed by five words or phrases lettered A through E. Choose the lettered word or phrase that is *most nearly* OPPOSITE in meaning to the word in capital letters. *PRINT THE LETTER OF THE CORRECT ANSWER IN THE SPACE AT THE RIGHT.*

TEST 1

1. ABEYANCE — A. revival B. following orders C. temporary inactivity D. adjournment E. concealment   1. ...
2. ACADEMIC — A. unseasoned B. scholarly C. practical D. attainable E. superficial   2. ...
3. AFFECTATION — A. histrionics B. conquetry C. shield D. airs E. ingeniousness   3. ...
4. AFFILIATE — A. thread B. honor C. cut away D. associate oneself E. feign   4. ...
5. ALLEGE — A. deny B. declare C. arouse D. arrest E. conjure   5. ...
6. ALLEVIATE — A. moderate B. assign C. tax D. antagonize E. deceive   6. ...
7. ANIMOSITY — A. hatred B. affection C. sprightliness D. animalism E. contempt   7. ...
8. APATHY — A. hatred B. indifference C. policy D. cowardice E. fervor   8. ...
9. APPAL — A. pierce B. apportion C. dismay D. attach E. gratify   9. ...
10. AUTHENTIC — A. severe B. gracious C. mendacious D. reliable E. supreme   10. ...
11. BRISK — A. large B. fragile C. alert D. flagging E. tolerant   11. ...
12. BRUSQUE — A. keen B. smooth C. menacing D. quick E. abrupt   12. ...
13. CALUMNIOUS — A. disastrous B. quartz-like C. laudatory E. slanderous E. querulous   13. ...
14. CANDID — A. straightforward B. evasive C. profound D. pleasant E. contrite   14. ...
15. CAROUSE — A. cajole B. revel C. decay D. induce E. abstain   15. ...
16. CELIBATE — A. chaste B. spouseless C. pertaining to funerals D. relic E. conjugal   16. ...
17. CLEMENCY — A. weather condition B. climbing plant C. type of cloud D. rigor E. mercy   17. ...
18. COMMODIOUS — A. inutile B. spacious C. ordinary D. interchangeable E. useful   18. ...
19. COMPETENT — A. equivalent B. compact C. adequate D. based on rivalry E. maladroit   19. ...
20. COMPLICITY — A. deceit B. antipathy C. partnership in wrong D. collusion E. delight in society   20. ...
21. CONSTERNATION — A. dissapointment B. dismay C. disapproval D. distrust E. intrepidity   21. ...
22. CONTAMINATE — A. include B. expurgate C. pollute D. adjacent E. reflect upon   22. ...
23. CORROBORATE — A. withdraw B. terminate C. disavow D. confirm E. correlate   23. ...
24. COSMIC — A. funny B. vast C. greasy D. childish E. finite   24. ...
25. CRITERION — A. standard B. anomaly C. judgment D. analysis E. probability   25. ...

TEST 2

1. CRUCIAL — A. pending B. conditional C. critical D. unreasonable E. unessential   1. ...
2. CULPABILITY — A. misprint B. blame C. felony D. impeccability E. whitewash   2. ...
3. DAUB — A. alarm B. delay C. depict D. stupefy E. smear   3. ...
4. DELINEATE — A. crack B. blotch C. do twice D. make of linen E. describe   4. ...
5. DEVIATING — A. conspiring B. depressing C. indirect D. unswerving E. turning   5. ...
6. DILAPIDATED — A. lonely B. integral C. ruined D. sequestered E. old-fashioned   6. ...
7. DILATORY — A. reclining B. spiteful C. expeditious D. praiseworthy E. procrastinating   7. ...
8. DISPATCH — A. curb B. argue C. send off D. mend E. receive   8. ...
9. DOCILE — A. parasitic B. ungovernable C. mournful D. teachable E. compliant   9. ...
10. DRIFT — A. meaning B. tendency C. riot D. motion E. procession   10. ...
11. DUALITY — A. unity B. falsity C. biformity D. perversity E. intactness   11. ...
12. DUBIOUS — A. questionable B. categorical C. sufficient D. pleasant to the ear E. composed   12. ...
13. DURABLE — A. flimsy B. permanent C. ugly D. timely E. callous   13. ...
14. ECCENTRIC — A. peculiar B. convergent C. ecliptic D. eclectic E. pragmatic   14. ...
15. EMBELLISH — A. defraud B. deface C. represent symbolically D. point up E. review   15. ...
16. EMBRYONIC — A. accelerated B. many-colored C. rudimentary D. undeveloped E. perfected   16. ...
17. ENIGMATIC — A. cognitive B. fraudulent C. odious D. magical E. puzzling   17. ...
18. EPIGRAMMATIC — A. pointed B. national C. ungrammatical D. scabrous E. concise   18. ...
19. FANATICISM — A. perplexity B. indifference C. endurance D. flatulence E. excessive enthusiasm   19. ...
20. FORMIDABLE — A. menacing B. conventional C. loathsome D. apprehensive E. resolute   20. ...
21. GAWKY — A. gaudy B. clumsy C. meager D. elegant E. straightforward   21. ...
22. GENESIS — A. gender B. origin C. outcome D. inception E. exodus   22. ...
23. HILARITY — A. celerity B. mirth C. despondence D. abandon E. covetousness   23. ...
24. HOSTILE — A. singular B. convincing C. poisonous D. stimulating E. amicable   24. ...
25. HYBRID — A. mongrel B. eugenic C. exaggerated D. dwarfed E. homogenous   25. ...

TEST 3

1. IMPEDIMENT — A. accusation B. hindrance C. succor D. admission E. inhibition   1. ...
2. IMPERVIOUS — A. incomparable B. impenetrable C. inhuman D. trackless D. dissoluble   2. ...
3. INCREDIBLE — A. hard to believe B. skeptical C. bad beyond correction D. indisputable D. illogical   3. ...

Test 3/4

4. INGENIOUS   A. frank B. deceitful C. ingenuous   4. ...
                  D. subversive E. clever
5. INTEGRITY   A. honesty B. opprobrium C. humor D. courage 5. ...
                  E. knowledge
6. INTIMIDATE   A. to defy B. to make afraid C. to come with- 6. ...
                  out invitation D. to weary E. to make less fearful
7. INTROSPECTION A. bending backwards B. insertion C. performa- 7. ...
                  tion D. self examination E. extroversion
8. JOSTLE   A. trip B. elbow C. bully D. rob E. quail   8. ...
9. LAVISH   A. niggardly B. extravagant C. prodigal   9. ...
                  D. convalescent E. plain
10. LENIENCY   A. transparent substance B. stringency   10. ...
                  C. fickleness D. forbearance E. decay
11. MERCENARY   A. egoistic B. pestilential C. altruistic   11. ...
                  D. greedy E. venal
12. MEDIOCRE   A. yellow B. boundless C. ordinary E. eminent 12. ...
                  E. tiny
13. NOVELTY   A. modernism B. pseudonym C. relic D. innova- 13. ...
                  tion E. quaintness
14. OBSOLETE   A. antiquated B. polite C. neglected   14. ...
                  D. rectangular E. vernal
15. ONSLAUGHT   A. furious attack B. murder C. repulse   15. ...
                  D. adventure E. severe punishment
16. OUST   A. evict B. banish C. injure D. admit   16. ...
                  E. cry out
17. PALATABLE   A. toothsome B. savory C. soft D. intoler-   17. ...
                  able E. vindictive
18. PALLID   A. wretched B. funereal C. ghastly D. spectral 18. ...
                  E. vivid
19. PALTRY   A. consequential B. pitiable C. grandiloquent 19. ...
                  D. prevalent E. petty
20. PARABLE   A. analogy B. pattern C. phenomenon D. fable 20. ...
                  E. allegory
21. PARAPHRASE   A. restate B. convey C. reword D. articulate 21. ...
                  E. translate
22. PARCH   A. swab B. saturate C. desiccate D. sponge   22. ...
                  E. scorch
23. PATHOLOGICAL A. morbid B. virulent C. salubrious E. diseased 23. ...
                  E. implied
24. PERMEATE   A. enfilade B. traverse C. pervade D. infil- 24. ...
                  trate E. block
25. PERPETUATE   A. obliterate B. punish C. preserve D. flourish 25. ...
                  E. enshrine

TEST 4

1. PERTINENT   A. appropriate B. awkward C. obstinate   1. ...
                  D. abusive E. irrelevant
2. PONDER   A. reflect B. hazard C. argue D. reject   2. ...
                  E. consider
3. POLLUTE   A. spread B. foul C. stain D. decontaminate   3. ...
                  E. rebut
4. POSTHUMOUS   A. hastily B. extant C. inappropriate   4. ...
                  D. happening after one's death E. unawakened

5. PREDILECTION   A. maintenance B. negotiation C. investment   5. ...
                  D. inclination E. evulsion
6. PRETEXT   A. reason B. fact C. excuse D. opinion   6. ...
                  E. illusion
7. PRODIGAL   A. perturbing B. wasteful C. venal D. large   7. ...
                  E. wandering
8. REFUTE   A. disobey B. disprove C. remove D. affirm   8. ...
                  E. strike out
9. RELENTLESS   A. compassionate B. unmoved by pity C. confident 9. ...
                  D. unexciting E. graceful
10. RETICENT   A. backward B. rash C. timid D. reserved   10. ...
                  E. gushing
11. SEDENTARY   A. soothing B. calm C. migratory D. aged   11. ...
                  E. stationary
12. SKEPTICISM   A. cynicism B. simplicity C. critical state of 12. ...
                  mind D. distortion E. chariness
13. SMUG   A. uncomplaisant B. adjacent C. self-satisfied 13. ...
                  D. hazy E. cozy
14. SPASMODIC   A. continuous B. intermittent C. feverish   14. ...
                  D. gradual E. momentary
15. STILTED   A. formal B. subdued C. deprived D. archaic   15. ...
                  E. facile
16. SUCCINCT   A. superfluous B. concise C. pithy D. succu-   16. ...
                  lent E. colloquial
17. SURREPTITIOUS A. stealthy B. surprising C. authorized   17. ...
                  D. affected E. unobserved
18. SUSCEPTIBLE   A. aggressive B. impotent C. cowering   18. ...
                  D. unimpressionable E. hesitant
19. TANTRUM   A. symbol B. tranquility C. commiseration   19. ...
                  D. conundrum E. display of temper
20. TATTERS   A. finery B. gossip C. sails D. riches E. rags 20. ...

KEYS (CORRECT ANSWERS)

	TEST 1			TEST 2			TEST 3			TEST 4	
1.	A	11. D	1.	E	11. A	1.	C	11. C	1.	E	11. C
2.	E	12. B	2.	D	12. B	2.	E	12. D	2.	B	12. B
3.	E	13. C	3.	C	13. A	3.	D	13. C	3.	D	13. A
4.	C	14. B	4.	B	14. D	4.	C	14. E	4.	B	14. A
5.	A	15. E	5.	D	15. B	5.	B	15. C	5.	E	15. E
6.	D	16. E	6.	B	16. E	6.	A	16. D	6.	B	16. A
7.	B	17. D	7.	C	17. A	7.	E	17. D	7.	C	17. C
8.	E	18. A	8.	A	18. E	8.	E	18. E	8.	D	18. D
9.	E	19. E	9.	B	19. B	9.	A	19. A	9.	A	19. B
10.	C	20. B	10.	E	20. B	10.	B	20. C	10.	E	20. A
	21. E			21. D			21. E				
	22. B			22. C			22. B				
	23. C			23. C			23. C				
	24. E			24. E			24. E				
	25. B			25. E			25. A				

ANTONYMS/OPPOSITES
EXAMINATION SECTION
TEST 1

DIRECTIONS: Each question below consists of a word printed in capital letters, followed by five words or phrases lettered A through E. Choose the lettered word or phrase that is *most nearly* OPPOSITE in meaning to the word in capital letters. *PRINT THE LETTER OF THE CORRECT ANSWER IN THE SPACE AT THE RIGHT.*

1. CELERITY   1.____
   - A. torpor
   - B. felicity
   - C. fame
   - D. acrimony
   - E. temerity

2. APATHETIC   2.____
   - A. stoical
   - B. amative
   - C. lissome
   - D. finical
   - E. redolent

3. FLACCID   3.____
   - A. cold
   - B. sterile
   - C. brave
   - D. stiff
   - E. whimsical

4. INGENUOUS   4.____
   - A. foolish
   - B. intelligent
   - C. wily
   - D. indigent
   - E. native

5. AMENABLE   5.____
   - A. prayerful
   - B. conciliatory
   - C. pliant
   - D. truculent
   - E. mendacious

6. PARSIMONIOUS   6.____
   - A. benevolent
   - B. worldly
   - C. scoffing
   - D. ungrammatical
   - E. grudging

7. INDIGENOUS   7.____
   - A. caustic
   - B. factitious
   - C. exotic
   - D. opulent
   - E. sophisticated

8. SAPIENT   8.____
   - A. distasteful
   - B. animalistic
   - C. ignorant
   - D. jejune
   - E. zestful

9. TENUOUS   9.____
   - A. substantial
   - B. decadent
   - C. salubrious
   - D. illogical
   - E. slender

10. ZENITH   10.____
    - A. acme
    - B. nadir
    - C. pentacle
    - D. azimuth
    - E. apogee

11. RESTIVE
    A. overactive   B. refractory   C. compliant
    D. uneasy   E. listless

12. ADAMANT
    A. primeval   B. laudatory   C. polite
    D. yielding   E. intractable

13. DISCRETE
    A. continuous   B. separate   C. foolish
    D. tactful   E. serrated

14. SANGUINE
    A. bloody   B. diffident   C. happy
    D. pale   E. confident

15. PLACATE
    A. retaliate   B. confuse   C. wander
    D. nettle   E. condone

16. FATUOUS
    A. inane   B. stout   C. witty
    D. empty   E. vacuous

17. INNOCUOUS
    A. toxic   B. guileful   C. gullible
    D. criminal   E. culpable

18. DEARTH
    A. demise   B. copiousness   C. nativity
    D. distaste   E. lack

19. RESPITE
    A. affirmation   B. intermission C. continuance
    D. colloquy   E. fairness

20. LACONIC
    A. turgid   B. replete   C. tearful
    D. negligent   E. draconic

21. ANIMADVERSION
    A. censure   B. distaste   C. spirituality
    D. bestiality   E. approbation

22. NOISOME
    A. boisterous   B. beneficial   C. villous
    D. pallid   E. noxious

23. EXPURGATE   23.____

    A. cleanse   B. harden   C. improve
    D. deflect   E. smirch

24. ATAVISM   24.____

    A. progression   B. favoritism   C. inclination
    D. cannibalism   E. reversion

25. ATTRITION   25.____

    A. appeasement   B. capitulation   C. wearing away
    D. calming down   E. aggrandizement

KEYS (CORRECT ANSWERS)

1. A		11. C	
2. B		12. D	
3. D		13. A	
4. C		14. B	
5. D		15. D	
6. A		16. C	
7. C		17. A	
8. C		18. B	
9. A		19. C	
10. B		20. A	

21. E
22. B
23. E
24. A
25. E

TEST 2

DIRECTIONS: Each question below consists of a word printed in capital letters, followed by five words or phrases lettered A through E. Choose the lettered word or phrase that is *most nearly* OPPOSITE in meaning to the word in capital letters. *PRINT THE LETTER OF THE CORRECT ANSWER IN THE SPACE AT THE RIGHT*

1. FABRICATE
   - A. consume
   - B. furrow
   - C. construct
   - D. materialize
   - E. delete

   1.___

2. COMMAND
   - A. mandate
   - B. consummation
   - C. correlation
   - D. commitment
   - E. supplication

   2.___

3. DISSIPATE
   - A. sip
   - B. amass
   - C. disturb
   - D. outdistance
   - E. disperse

   3.___

4. UNBIASED
   - A. unfair
   - B. unreasonable
   - C. uniform
   - D. equitable
   - E. disquieting

   4.___

5. SATURNINE
   - A. buoyant
   - B. gloomy
   - C. aspiring
   - D. incongruous
   - E. splenetic

   5.___

6. PROFITABLE
   - A. preferable
   - B. chagrined
   - C. ruinous
   - D. lucrative
   - E. profligate

   6.___

7. GENERATING
   - A. generous
   - B. originating
   - C. degenerating
   - D. terminating
   - E. ingenuous

   7.___

8. SANCTION
   - A. safety
   - B. performance
   - C. injunction
   - D. sanctuary
   - E. permission

   8.___

9. PROBABLE
   - A. perchance
   - B. imprudent
   - C. unlikely
   - D. perilous
   - E. unsavory

   9.___

10. FRUITION
    - A. exposure
    - B. harvest
    - C. frustration
    - D. neglect
    - E. attainment

    10.___

102

11. RANCOROUS 11._____
   A. benign   B. confusing   C. satiated
   D. complex   E. malicious

12. AVARICIOUS 12._____
   A. munificent   B. rapacious   C. analogous
   D. perverse   E. atonal

13. UNIQUE 13._____
   A. uniform   B. single   C. utilitarian
   D. senescent   E. unitary

14. PROCURE 14._____
   A. decline   B. reap   C. forfeit
   D. effect   E. contrive

15. RAVENOUS 15._____
   A. birdlike   B. hungry   C. rancid
   D. venial   E. sated

16. INNOCUOUS 16._____
   A. mixed   B. pernicious   C. defiled
   D. harmless   E. diffused

17. PERMEATE 17._____
   A. smooth   B. pulverize   C. obstruct
   D. pollute   E. penetrate

18. AXIOM 18._____
   A. adage   B. proof   C. precept
   D. dictum   E. hearsay

19. RELEVANT 19._____
   A. immaterial   B. pertinent   C. relenting
   D. capable   E. released

20. POTENT 20._____
   A. secretive   B. powerful   C. restive
   D. puissant   E. enervated

21. AMELIORATE 21._____
   A. improve   B. embitter   C. alter
   D. mellow   E. impair

22. IMPENDING 22._____
   A. pendulous   B. impeding   C. fortuitous
   D. imminent   E. looming

23. LATENT

    A. tricky   B. hidden   C. pompous
    D. overt   E. hateful

24. DISCERNMENT

    A. concern   B. obtuseness   C. distance
    D. sickness   E. acumen

25. SUAVE

    A. genuine   B. captive   C. gauche
    D. bland   E. captious

KEYS (CORRECT ANSWERS)

1.	A		11.	A
2.	E		12.	A
3.	B		13.	A
4.	A		14.	C
5.	A		15.	E
6.	C		16.	B
7.	D		17.	C
8.	C		18.	E
9.	C		19.	A
10.	C		20.	E

21. B
22. C
23. D
24. B
25. C

TEST 3

DIRECTIONS: Each question below consists of a word printed in capital letters, followed by five words or phrases lettered A through E. Choose the lettered word or phrase that is *most nearly* OPPOSITE in meaning to the word in capital letters. *PRINT THE LETTER OF THE CORRECT ANSWER IN THE SPACE AT THE RIGHT.*

1. WORLDLY 1.____
   - A. trifling
   - B. secular
   - C. mundane
   - D. unworthy
   - E. impractical

2. BEG 2.____
   - A. seek
   - B. implore
   - C. convert
   - D. vaunt
   - E. donate

3. ERUDITE 3.____
   - A. impolite
   - B. learned
   - C. correct
   - D. illiterate
   - E. contrite

4. CURSORY 4.____
   - A. protracted
   - B. persistent
   - C. evanescent
   - D. superficial
   - E. gentle

5. ENIGMATIC 5.____
   - A. evident
   - B. enormous
   - C. lucid
   - D. abstruse
   - E. sphinxlike

6. PROSCRIBE 6.____
   - A. banish
   - B. condemn
   - C. diagnose poorly
   - D. transcend
   - E. prescribe

7. TURBID 7.____
   - A. limpid
   - B. muddy
   - C. moody
   - D. settled
   - E. turgid

8. PERSPICACITY 8.____
   - A. keenness
   - B. penetration
   - C. rudeness
   - D. discernment
   - E. insensibility

9. CONTIGUOUS 9.____
   - A. contagious
   - B. adjoining
   - C. intolerant
   - D. unconnected
   - E. uncontaminated

10. ASSUAGE 10.____
    - A. intensify
    - B. coagulate
    - C. alleviate
    - D. congeal
    - E. molest

11. PROTAGONIST
    A. enemy   B. participant   C. champion
    D. protector   E. patron

12. VIRULENT
    A. vehement   B. virtuous   C. deadly
    D. reparatory   E. virile

13. PROLIX
    A. tiresome   B. exciting   C. wordy
    D. terse   E. pompous

14. LEVITY
    A. lengthiness   B. glumness   C. lenience
    D. frivolity   E. lewdness

15. METICULOUS
    A. careful   B. approximate   C. untrue
    D. metallic   E. indiscriminate

16. ANALOGOUS
    A. tantamount   B. extracurricular C. distinctive
    D. presumptuous E. cavernous

17. VICARIOUS
    A. inconsiderate B. direct   C. fraudulent
    D. substitute   E. prestigious

18. ABROGATION
    A. promulgation B. repeal   C. extension
    D. investigation E. postponement

19. HOMOGENEOUS
    A. manly   B. assorted   C. creamy
    D. similar   E. parallel

20. ARRAIGN
    A. accuse   B. convict   C. disentangle
    D. disarrange   E. discharge

21. ABJURE
    A. remove   B. disavow   C. acknowledge
    D. imagine   E. entreat

22. INTESTATE
    A. relating to inner parts   B. legally devised   C. shipped from one place to another
    D. subject to taxation   E. not disposed of by will

23. ANCILLARY	23.____

    A. deterrent   B. temporary   C. auxiliary
    D. approved   E. additional

24. EXTRANEOUS	24.____

    A. foreign   B. accidental   C. mixed
    D. indigenous   E. adventitious

25. DISPARAGE	25.____

    A. divide   B. dismiss   C. depreciate
    D. discourage   E. dignify

KEYS (CORRECT ANSWERS)

1. E		11. A	
2. E		12. D	
3. D		13. D	
4. A		14. B	
5. C		15. E	
6. E		16. C	
7. A		17. B	
8. E		18. A	
9. D		19. B	
10. A		20. E	

21. C
22. B
23. A
24. D
25. E

TEST 4

DIRECTIONS: Each question below consists of a word printed in capital letters, followed by five words or phrases lettered A through E. Choose the lettered word or phrase that is *most nearly* OPPOSITE in meaning to the word in capital letters. *PRINT THE LETTER OF THE CORRECT ANSWER IN THE SPACE AT THE RIGHT.*

1. FUGACIOUS
   - A. pugnacious
   - B. tenacious
   - C. mendacious
   - D. settled
   - E. migratory

1.___

2. THRASONICAL
   - A. treasonable
   - B. gingival
   - C. vainglorious
   - D. unassuming
   - E. lyrical

2.___

3. PELAGIC
   - A. terrestrial
   - B. aquatic
   - C. noncontagious
   - D. polemical
   - E. epigrammatic

3.___

4. FUSCOUS
   - A. importunate
   - B. chaste
   - C. radiant
   - D. fractious
   - E. amenable

4.___

5. CREPUSCULAR
   - A. glimmering
   - B. crackling
   - C. pussy
   - D. mutable
   - E. distinct

5.___

6. NOISOME
   - A. attractive
   - B. noxious
   - C. inoffensive
   - D. winsome
   - E. noiseless

6.___

7. PEJORATIVE
   - A. appreciative
   - B. acceding
   - C. ultimate
   - D. alliterative
   - E. conceding

7.___

8. JEJUNE
   - A. valiant
   - B. vital
   - C. graceful
   - D. senile
   - E. incipient

8.___

9. FULGENT
   - A. divergent
   - B. lambent
   - C. unresplendent
   - D. cogent
   - E. indigent

9.___

10. LENITIVE
    - A. laxative
    - B. provocative
    - C. menial
    - D. incursive
    - E. malevolent

10.___

108

11. IRREFRAGABLE

    A. breakable   B. desirable   C. tractable
    D. inconclusive   E. refutable

12. INCHOATE

    A. chaotic   B. disclosed   C. coherent
    D. infatuated   E. complete

13. MINATORY

    A. vanishing   B. nugatory   C. myriad
    D. malignant   E. propitious

14. AMBIENT

    A. wandering   B. pandering   C. transient
    D. remote   E. hostile

15. EUPHEMISTIC

    A. euphuistic   B. grating   C. masochistic
    D. palpable   E. insolent

16. FACTIOUS

    A. fractious   B. fictitious   C. scrupulous
    D. seemly   E. disinterested

17. FRIABLE

    A. unseasoned   B. palatable   C. renascent
    D. indestructible E. adhesive

18. HEGEMONY

    A. thraldom   B. testimony   C. followership
    D. necromancy   E. obligation

19. IMMANENT

    A. illative   B. imminent   C. emanating
    D. unessential   E. clement

20. INDEFEASIBLE

    A. defensible   B. abrogable   C. disputable
    D. deferential   E. execrable

21. EQUIVOCAL

    A. ambiguous   B. ambivalent   C. equitable
    D. esoteric   E. unquestionable

22. LIVID

    A. lurid   B. discolored   C. unrestrained
    D. rubicund   E. ghastly

23. MOIETY

    A. impiety   B. notoriety   C. unity
    D. harmony   E. inconsistency

24. PEREMPTORY

    A. dogmatic   B. authoritarian   C. indecisive
    D. conciliatory   E. whimsical

25. VENIAL

    A. mercenary   B. venous   C. purulent
    D. aberrant   E. loathsome

KEYS (CORRECT ANSWERS)

1.	D		11.	E
2.	D		12.	E
3.	A		13.	E
4.	C		14.	D
5.	E		15.	B
6.	C		16.	E
7.	A		17.	D
8.	B		18.	A
9.	C		19.	D
10.	B		20.	B

21. E
22. D
23. C
24. C
25. E

TESTS IN SENTENCE COMPLETION / 1 BLANK
EXAMINATION SECTION
TEST 1

DIRECTIONS: Each question in this section consists of a sentence in which one word is missing; a blank line indicates where the word has been removed from the sentence. Beneath each sentence are five words, *one* of which is the missing word. You are to select the letter of the missing word by deciding which one of the five words BEST fits in with the meaning of the sentence. *PRINT THE LETTER OF THE CORRECT ANSWER IN THE SPACE AT THE RIGHT.*

1. A man who cannot win honor in his own _____ will have a very small chance of winning it from posterity.

    A. right   B. field   C. country   D. way   E. age

2. The latent period for the contractile response to direct stimulation of the muscle has quite another and shorte value, encompassing only a utilization period. Hence it is that the term *latent period* must be _____ carefully each time that it is used.

    A. checked   B. timed   C. introduced
    D. defined   E. selected

3. Many television watchers enjoy stories which contain violence. Consequently those television producers who are dominated by rating systems aim to _____ the popular taste.

    A. raise   B. control   C. gratify   D. ignore   E. lower

4. No other man loses so much, so _____, so absolutely, as the beaten candidate for high public office.

    A. bewilderingly   B. predictably   C. disgracefully
    D. publicly   E. cheerfully

5. Mathematics is the product of thought operating by means of _____ for the purpose of expressing general laws.

    A. reasoning   B. symbols   C. words
    D. examples   E. science

6. Deductive reasoning is that form of reasoning in which the conclusion must necessarily follow if we accept the premise as true. In deduction, it is _____ the premise to be true and the conclusion false.

    A. impossible   B. inevitable   C. reasonable
    D. surprising   E. unlikely

7. Because in the administration it hath respect not to the group but to the _____, our form of government is called a democracy.

    A. courts   B. people   C. majority
    D. individual   E. law

8. Before criticizing the work of an artist one needs to _____ the artist's purpose. 8.____

    A. understand   B. reveal   C. defend
    D. correct   E. change

9. Their work was commemorative in character and consisted largely of _____ erected upon the occasion of victories. 9.____

    A. towers   B. tombs   C. monuments
    D. castles   E. fortresses

10. Every good story is carefully contrived: the elements of the story are _____ to fit with one another in order to make an effect on the reader. 10.____

    A. read   B. learned   C. emphasized
    D. reduced   E. planned

KEY (CORRECT ANSWERS)

1. E   6. A
2. D   7. D
3. C   8. A
4. D   9. C
5. B   10. E

TEST 2

DIRECTIONS: Each question in this section consists of a sentence in which one word is missing; a blank line indicates where the word has been removed from the sentence. Beneath each sentence are five words, *one* of which is the missing word. You are to select the letter of the missing word by deciding which one of the five words BEST fits in with the meaning of the sentence. *PRINT THE LETTER OF THE CORRECT ANSWER IN THE SPACE AT THE RIGHT.*

1. One of the most prevalent erroneous contentions is that Argentina is a country of _____ agricultural resources and needs only the arrival of ambitious settlers.   1._____
   - A. modernized
   - B. flourishing
   - C. undeveloped
   - D. waning
   - E. limited

2. The last official statistics for the town indicated the presence of 24,212 Italians, 6,450 Magyars, and 2,315 Germans, which ensures to the _____ a numerical preponderance.   2._____
   - A. Germans
   - B. figures
   - C. town
   - D. Magyars
   - E. Italians

3. Precision of wording is necessary in good writing; by choosing words that exactly convey the desired meaning, one can avoid _____.   3._____
   - A. duplicity
   - B. incongruity
   - C. complexity
   - D. ambiguity
   - E. implications

4. Various civilians of the liberal school in the British Parliament remonstrated that there were no grounds for _____ of French aggression, since the Emperor showed less disposition to augment the navy than had Louis Philippe.   4._____
   - A. suppression
   - B. retaliation
   - C. apprehension
   - D. concealment
   - E. commencement

5. _____ is as clear and definite as any of our urges; we wonder what is in a sealed letter or what is being said in a telephone booth.   5._____
   - A. Envy
   - B. Curiosity
   - C. Knowledge
   - D. Communication
   - E. Ambition

6. It is a rarely philosophic soul who can make a _____ the other alternative forever into the limbo of forgotten things.   6._____
   - A. mistake
   - B. wish
   - C. change
   - D. choice
   - E. plan

7. A creditor is worse than a master. A master owns only your person, but a creditor owns your _____ as well.   7._____
   - A. aspirations
   - B. potentialities
   - C. ideas
   - D. dignity
   - E. wealth

8. People _____ small faults, in order to insinuate that they have no great ones.   8._____
   - A. create
   - B. display
   - C. confess
   - D. seek
   - E. reject

9. Andrew Jackson believed that wars were inevitable, and to him the length and irregularity of our coast presented a _____ that called for a more than merely passive navy.

    A. defense   B. barrier   C. provocation
    D. vulnerability   E. dispute

10. The progressive yearly _____ of the land, caused by the depositing of mud from the river, makes it possible to estimate the age of excavated remains by noting the depth at which they are found below the present level of the valley.

    A. erosion   B. elevation   C. improvement
    D. irrigation   E. displacement

KEY (CORRECT ANSWERS)

1. C   6. D
2. E   7. D
3. D   8. C
4. C   9. D
5. B   10. B

TEST 3

DIRECTIONS: Each question in this section consists of a sentence in which one word is missing; a blank line indicates where the word has been removed from the sentence. Beneath each sentence are five words, *one* of which is the missing word. You are to select the letter of the missing word by deciding which one of the five words BEST fits in with the meaning of the sentence. *PRINT THE LETTER OF THE CORRECT ANSWER IN THE SPACE AT THE RIGHT.*

1. The judge exercised commendable _____ dismissing the charge against the prisoner. In spite of the clamor that surrounded the trial, and the heinousness of the offense, the judge could not be swayed to overlook the lack of facts in the case.   1.____

    A. avidity B. meticulousness C. clemency
    D. balance E. querulousness

2. The pianist played the concerto _____, displaying such facility and skill as has rarely been matched in this old auditorium.   2.____

    A. strenuous B. spiritedly C. passionately
    D. casually E. deftly

3. The Tanglewood Symphony Orchestra holds its outdoor concerts far from city turmoil in a _____, bucolic setting.   3.____

    A. spectacular B. atavistic C. serene
    D. chaotic E. catholic

4. Honest satire gives true joy to the thinking man. Thus, the satirist is most _____ when he points out the hypocrisy in human actions.   4.____

    A. elated B. humiliated C. ungainly
    D. repressed E. disdainful

5. She was a(n) _____ preferred the company of her books to the pleasures of cafe society.   5.____

    A. philanthropist B. stoic C. exhibitionist
    D. extrovert E. introvert

6. So many people are so convinced that people are driven by _____ motives that they cannot believe that anybody is unselfish!   6.____

    A. interior B. ulterior C. unworth
    D. selfish E. destructive

7. These _____ results were brought about by a chain of fortuitous events.   7.____

    A. unfortunate B. odd C. harmful
    D. haphazard E. propitious

8. The bank teller's _____ of the funds was discovered the following month when the auditors examined the books.   8.____

    A. embezzlement B. burglary C. borrowing
    D. assignment E. theft

9. The monks gathered in the _____ for their evening meal.   9.____

   A. lounge   B. auditorium   C. refectory
   D. rectory   E. solarium

10. Local officials usually have the responsibility in each area of determining when the need   10.____
    is sufficiently great to _____ withdrawals from the community water supply.

    A. encourage   B. justify   C. discontinue
    D. advocate   E. forbid

KEY (CORRECT ANSWERS)

1. D   6. B
2. E   7. D
3. C   8. A
4. A   9. C
5. E   10. B

TEST 4

DIRECTIONS: Each question in this section consists of a sentence in which one word is missing; a blank line indicates where the word has been removed from the sentence. Beneath each sentence are five words, *one* of which is the missing word. You are to select the letter of the missing word by deciding which one of the five words BEST fits in with the meaning of the sentence. *PRINT THE LETTER OF THE CORRECT ANSWER IN THE SPACE AT THE RIGHT*

1. The life of the mining camps as portrayed by Bret Harte—boisterous, material, brawling— was in direct _____ to the contemporary Eastern world of conventional morals and staid deportment depicted by other men of letters.
    - A. model
    - B. parallel
    - C. antithesis
    - D. relationship
    - E. response

2. The agreements were to remain in force for three years and were subject to automatic _____ unless terminated by the parties concerned on one month's notice.
    - A. renewal
    - B. abrogation
    - C. amendment
    - D. confiscation
    - E. option

3. In a democracy, people are recognized for what they do rather than for their _____.
    - A. alacrity
    - B. ability
    - C. reputation
    - D. skill
    - E. pedigree

4. Although he had often loudly proclaimed his _____ concerning world affairs, he actually read widely and was usually the best informed person in his circle.
    - A. weariness
    - B. complacency
    - C. condolence
    - D. indifference
    - E. worry

5. This student holds the _____ record of being the sole failure in his class.
    - A. flagrant
    - B. unhappy
    - C. egregious
    - D. dubious
    - E. unusual

6. She became enamored _____ acrobat when she witnessed his act.
    - A. of
    - B. with
    - C. for
    - D. by
    - E. about

7. This will _____ all previous wills.
    - A. abrogates
    - B. denies
    - C. supersedes
    - D. prevents
    - E. continues

8. In the recent terrible Chicago _____, over ninety children were found dead as a result of the fire.
    - A. hurricane
    - B. destruction
    - C. panic
    - D. holocaust
    - E. accident

9. I can ascribe no better reason why he shunned society than that he was a _____.
    - A. mentor
    - B. Centaur
    - C. aristocrat
    - D. misanthrope
    - E. failure

10. One who attempts to learn all the known facts before he comes to a conclusion may most aptly be described as a _____.   10._____

    A. realist
    B. philosopher
    C. cynic
    D. pessimist
    E. skeptic

KEY (CORRECT ANSWERS)

1. C
2. A
3. E
4. D
5. D

6. A
7. C
8. D
9. D
10. E

TEST 5

DIRECTIONS: Each question in this section consists of a sentence in which one word is missing; a blank line indicates where the word has been removed from the sentence. Beneath each sentence are five words, *one* of which is the missing word. You are to select the letter of the missing word by deciding which one of the five words BEST fits in with the meaning of the sentence. *PRINT THE LETTER OF THE CORRECT ANSWER IN THE SPACE AT THE RIGHT.*

1. The prime minister, fleeing from the rebels who had seized the government, sought _____ in the church.

    A. revenge   B. mercy   C. relief
    D. salvation   E. sanctuary

    1.____

2. It does not take us long to conclude that it is foolish to fight the _____, and that it is far wiser to accept it.

    A. inevitable   B. inconsequential   C. impossible
    D. choice   E. invasion

    2.____

3. _____ is usually defined as an excessively high rate of interest.

    A. Injustice   B. Perjury   C. Exorbitant
    D. Embezzlement   E. Usury

    3.____

4. "I ask you, gentlemen of the jury, to find this man guilty since I have _____ the charges brought about him."

    A. documented   B. questioned   C. revised
    D. selected   E. confused

    4.____

5. Although the critic was a close friend of the producer, he told him that he could not _____ his play.

    A. condemn   B. prefer   C. congratulate
    D. endorse   E. revile

    5.____

6. Knowledge of human nature and motivation is an important _____ in all areas of endeavor.

    A. object   B. incentive   C. opportunity
    D. asset   E. goal

    6.____

7. Numbered among the audience were kings, princes, dukes, and even a maharajah, all attempting to _____ another in the glitter of their habiliments and the number of their escorts.

    A. supersede   B. outdo   C. guide
    D. vanquish   E. equal

    7.____

8. There seems to be a widespread feeling that peoples who are located below us in respect to latitude are _____ also in respect to intellect and ability.

    A. superior   B. melodramatic   C. inferior
    D. ulterior   E. contemptible

    8.____

119

9. This should be considered a(n) _____ rather than the usual occurrence.

    A. coincidence   B. specialty   C. development
    D. outgrowth   E. mirage

10. Those who were considered states' rights adherents in the early part of our history, espoused the diminution of the powers of the national government because they had always been _____ of these powers.

    A. solicitous   B. advocates   C. apprehensive
    D. mindful   E. respectful

KEY (CORRECT ANSWERS)

1. E	6. D
2. A	7. B
3. E	8. C
4. A	9. A
5. D	10. C

TEST 6

DIRECTIONS: Each question in this section consists of a sentence in which one word is missing; a blank line indicates where the word has been removed from the sentence. Beneath each sentence are five words, *one* of which is the missing word. You are to select the letter of the missing word by deciding which one of the five words BEST fits in with the meaning of the sentence. *PRINT THE LETTER OF THE CORRECT ANSWER IN THE SPACE AT THE RIGHT.*

1. We can see in retrospect that the high hopes for lasting peace conceived at Versailles in 1919 were _____. 1.____

   A. ingenuous B. transient C. nostalgic
   D. ingenious E. specious

2. One of the constructive effects of Nazism was the passage by the U.N. of a resolution to combat _____. 2.____

   A. armaments B. nationalism C. colonialism
   D. genocide E. geriatrics

3. In our prisons, the role of _____ often gains for certain inmates a powerful position among their fellow prisoners. 3.____

   A. informer B. clerk C. warden D. trusty E. turnkey

4. It is the _____ liar, experienced in the ways of the world, who finally trips upon some incongruous detail. 4.____

   A. consummate B. incorrigible C. congenital
   D. lagrant E. contemptible

5. Anyone who is called a misogynist can hardly be expected to look upon women with _____ contemptuous eyes. 5.____

   A. more than B. nothing less than C. decidedly
   D. other than E. always

6. Demagogues such as Hitler and Mussolini aroused the masses by appealing to their _____ rather than to their intellect. 6.____

   A. emotions B. reason C. nationalism
   D. conquests E. duty

7. He was in great demand as an entertainer for his _____ abilities: he could sing, dance, tell a joke, or relate a story with equally great skill and facility. 7.____

   A. versatile B. logical C. culinary
   D. histrionic E. creative

8. The wise politician is aware that, next to knowing when to seize an opportunity, it is also important to know when to _____ an advantage. 8.____

   A. develop B. seek C. revise
   D. proclaim E. forego

9. Books on psychology inform us that the best way to break a bad habit is to _____ a new habit in its place.

   A. expel
   B. substitute
   C. conceal
   D. curtail
   E. supplant

10. The author who uses one word where another uses a whole paragraph, should be considered a _____ writer.

    A. successful
    B. grandiloquent
    C. experienced
    D. prolix
    E. succinct

KEY (CORRECT ANSWERS)

1. A
2. D
3. A
4. A
5. D
6. A
7. A
8. E
9. B
10. E

ARITHMETICAL REASONING
EXAMINATION SECTION
TEST 1

DIRECTIONS: Each question or incomplete statement is followed by several suggested answers or completions. Select the one that BEST answers the question or completes the statement. *PRINT THE LETTER OF THE CORRECT ANSWER IN THE SPACE AT THE RIGHT.*

1. The population of a city is, approximately, 7.85 million. The area is approximately 200 square miles. The number of thousand persons per square mile is
   A. 3.925   B. 39.25   C. 392.5   D. 39250

2. The longest straight line that can be drawn to connect two points on the circumference of a circle whose radius is 9 inches is
   A. 9 inches   B. 18 inches   C. 28.2753 inches   D. 4.5 inches

3. It is believed that every even number is the sum of two prime numbers. Two prime numbers whose sum is 32 are
   A. 7, 25   B. 22, 21   C. 13, 19   D. 17, 15

4. To divide a number by 3000, we should *move* the decimal point 3 places to the
   A. right and divide by 3
   B. left and divide by 3
   C. right and multiply by 3
   D. left and multiply by 3

5. The difference between the area of a rectangle 6 ft. by 4 ft. and the area of a square having the *same* perimeter is
   A. 1 sq. ft.   B. 2 sq. ft.   C. 4 sq. ft.   D. none of these

6. The ratio of 1/4 to 3/8 is the *same* as the ratio of
   A. 1 to 3   B. 2 to 3   C. 3 to 2   D. 3 to 4

7. If 7½ is divided by 1 1/5, the quotient is
   A. 6 1/4   B. 9   C. 7 1/10   D. 6 3/5

8. A farmer has a cylindrical metal tank for watering his stock. It is 10 ft. in diameter and 3 ft. deep. If one cubic foot contains about 7.5 gallons, the *approximate* capacity of the tank in gallons is
   A. 12   B. 225   C. 4   D. 1707

9. The fraction which fits in the following series, 1/2, 1/10, _____, 1/250, is
   A. 1/20   B. 1/100   C. 1/10   D. 1/50

10. In two years, $200 with interest compounded semi-annually at 4% will amount to
    A. $216.48   B. $233.92   C. $208   D. $216

SOLUTIONS TO ARITHMETICAL REASONING

1. Answer: (B) 39.25

   $$\frac{40,000}{20)\overline{8,000,000}}$$ (number of persons per square mile)(approximate population)

   Answer: 39.25 or (approximately) 40 (thousand persons per sq. mi.)

2. Answer: (B) 18 inches

   9" + 9" = 18 inches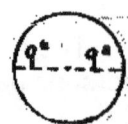

3. Answer: (C) 13, 19
   A prime number is an integer which cannot be divided by itself and one integer; a whole number as opposed to a fraction or a decimal.

4. Answer: (B) 3 places to the left and divide by

   $$\frac{2}{3)\overline{6,000.}}$$

5. Answer: (A) 1 sq. ft.

   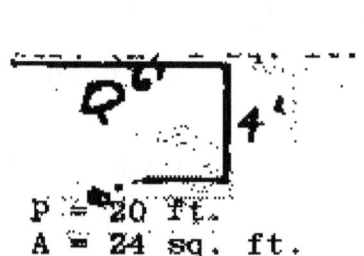
   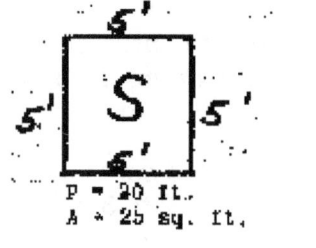

   P = 20 ft.   P = 20 ft.
   A = 24 sq.   A = 25 sq.

6. Answer: (B) 2 to 3

   $$\frac{1/4}{3/8} = 1/4 \div 3/8 = 1/4 \times 3/8 = 2/3$$

7. Answer: (A) 6 1/4

   $$\frac{7\,1/2}{1\,1/2} = \frac{15}{2} \div \frac{6}{5} = \frac{15}{2} \times \frac{5}{6} = \frac{25}{4} = 6\frac{1}{4}$$ OR $$1.2)\overline{7.5\,\tfrac{1}{4}} = 6\tfrac{3}{12}$$

3 (#1)

8. Answer: (B) 225

   $A = irR^2$
   $= 3(5)^2$
   = 75 sq. ft.

   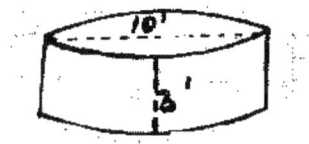

   ```
   225
   ×7.5
   ────
   1125
   1575    gal
   ──────
   1687.5
   ```

   Volume of tank = 75 × 3 = 225 cu. ft.
   (approximate capacity of tank in gallons)

9. Answer: (D) 1/50
   A geometric series: each number is multiplied by the same number to get the succeeding number. (Multiply each number by 1/5). ½, 1/10, 1/50/$216, 1/250. The missing number if 1/50.

10. Answer: (A) $216.48
    <u>Compound Interest</u>
    4% a year compounded semi-annually is the same as 2% for a half year

    A. $200 $200
        ×.02   × 4
        ─────   ─────
        $4.00 Interest for 1st half yr. $204 Principal for 1st half yr.

    B. $204 $204.00
        ×.02   × 4.08
        ─────   ───────
        $4.08 Interest for 2nd half yr. $208.08 Principal for 1st half of 2nd yr.

    C. $208.08 $208.08
        ×.02   × 4.16
        ──────   ───────
        $4.1616 Interest for 1st half of 2nd yr. $212.24 Principal for 2nd half of 2nd yr.

    D. $212.24 $212.24
        ×.02   × 4.24
        ──────   ───────
        $4.2448 Interest for 2nd half of 2nd yr. $216.48 Principal at end of 2nd half of 2nd yr.

TEST 2

DIRECTIONS: Each question or incomplete statement is followed by several suggested answers or completions. Select the one that BEST answers the question or completes the statement. *PRINT THE LETTER OF THE CORRECT ANSWER IN THE SPACE AT THE RIGHT.*

1. With a *tax rate* of .0200, a tax bill of $1050 corresponds to an *assessed valuation* of   1.____
   A. $21,000 B. $52,500 C. $21 D. $1029

2. A sales agent, after deducting his commission of 6%, remits $2491 to his principal. The SALE amounted to   2.____
   A. $2809 B. $2640 C. $2650 D. $2341.54

3. The percent equivalent of .0295 is   3.____
   A. 2.95% B. 29.5% C. .295% D. 295%

4. An angle of 105 degrees is a _____ angle.   4.____
   A. straight B. acute C. obtuse D. reflex

5. A quart is approximately sixty cubic inches. A cu. ft. of water weighs approximately sixty pounds. Therefore, a quart of water weights *approximately*   5.____
   A. 2 lbs. B. 3 lbs. C. 4 lbs. D. 5 lbs.

6. If the *same* number is added to both the numerator and the denominator of a proper fraction, the   6.____
   A. value of the fraction is decreased
   B. value of the fraction is increased
   C. value of the fraction is unchanged
   D. effect of the operation depends on the original fraction

7. The *lease common multiple* of 3, 8, 9, 12 is   7.____
   A. 36 B. 72 C. 108 D. 144

8. On a bill of $100, the *difference* between a discount of 30% and 20% and a discount of 40% and 10% is   8.____
   A. nothing B. $2 C. $20 D. 20%

9. 1/3 percent of a number is 24. The NUMBER is   9.____
   A. 8 B. 72 C. 800 D. 7200

10. The cost of importing five dozen china dinner sets, billed at $32 per set, and paying a duty of 40% is   10.____
    A. $224 B. $2688 C. $768 D. $1344

SOLUTIONS TO ARITHMETICAL REASONING

1. Answer: (B) $52,500
   0200x = $1050   2x = $105,000
   200x = $10,500,000   x = $52,500 (assessed valuation)

2. Answer: (C) $2650
   $2491 + .06x = x
   x = 2491 + .06x

	Proof	
1.00x - .06x = 2491	$2650	$2491
	× .06	+ 159
	$159.00	$2650

   .94x = 2491
   .94x = 249,100

   $2,650
   94)249,100

3. Answer: (A) 2.95% [.0295 = 2.95%)

4. Answer: (C) obtuse angle
   An obtuse angle is an angle greater than 90°.

5. Answer: (A) 2 lbs.
   A quart = 60 cu. in.
   60 lbs. = 1 cu. ft. (or 1728 cu. in.) (12×12×12)
            (Keep like units of measure together)
   60 lbs. = 1728 cu. in.
   1 lb. = 1728/60 = approximately .29 cu. in.
   If 29 cu. in. weighs 1 lb., then 60 cu. in. weighs 2 lbs. (approximately). Therefore, a quart weighs 2 lbs. (approximately).

6. Answer: (B) the value of the fraction is increased

   (1) Start with the fraction 2/3

   (2) $\frac{2+2}{3+2} = \frac{4}{5}$ (Adding 2 to the numerator and the denominator)

   (3) $\frac{3}{2} = \frac{10}{15}$

   (4) $\frac{4}{5} = \frac{12}{15}$

7. Answer: (B) 72
   Common multiple can be evenly divided by all the numbers. Lease common multiple: the lowest of these numbers.

8. Answer: (B) $2
   Formula: Step 1. Express percentages as decimals
              Step 2. Subtract each discount from *one*
              Step 3. Multiply all the results
              Step 4. Subtract the product from *one*

              Step 1. .3, .2 and .4, .1
              Step 2. .7, .8 and .6, .9
              Step 3. .7 × .8 = .56 (represents percent remaining after the discounts
                      .6 × .9 = .54   are taken)
              Step 4. 1.00   1.00
                      -.56   -.54
                       .44   .46

              Then, $100 × .02 = $2.00

9. Answer: (D) 7200

   $\frac{1}{300}x = 24$;   x = 24×300;   x = 7200

10. Answer: (B) $2688

    $32 $1920
    ×60   ×.40
    $1920 Cost of dinner sets before paying duty $768.00 Duty

    $1920
    + 768
    $2688 Cost of dinner sets *after* paying duty

TEST 3

DIRECTIONS: Each question or incomplete statement is followed by several suggested answers or completions. Select the one that BEST answers the question or completes the statement. *PRINT THE LETTER OF THE CORRECT ANSWER IN THE SPACE AT THE RIGHT.*

1. A motorist travels 120 miles to his destination at the average speed of 60 miles per hour and returns to the starting point at the average speed of 40 miles per hour. His *average speed* for the ENTIRE trip is _____ miles per hour.
   A. 53   B. 50   C. 48   D. 45

   1._____

2. A snapshot measures 2 1/2 inches by 1 7/8 inches. It is to be enlarged so that the longer dimension will be 4 inches. The length of the enlarged *shorter* dimension will be
   A. 2 1/2 inches   B. 3 3/8 inches   C. 3 inches   D. none of these

   2._____

3. The approximate distance is, in feet, that an object falls in t seconds when dropped from a height is obtained by use of the formula $s = 16t^2$. In 8 seconds, the object will fall
   A. 15,384 feet   B. 1,024 feet   C. 256 feet   D. none of these

   3._____

4. The PRODUCT of 75^3 and 75^7 is
   A. $(75)^{10}$ B. $(75)^{21}$ C. $(5,625)^{10}$ D. $(150)^{10}$

   4._____

5. The scale of a map is: 3/4 of an inch = 10 miles. If the distance on the map between two towns is 6 inches, the *actual* distance is
   A. 45 miles   B. 60 miles   C. 80 miles   D. none of these

   5._____

6. If $d = m \dfrac{50}{m}$, and m is a positive number which increases in value, d

   A. increases in value
   B. remains unchanged
   B. decreases in value
   D. fluctuates up and down in value

   6._____

7. From a piece of tin in the shape of a square 6 inches on a side, the largest possible circle is cut out.
   Of the following, the ratio of the area of the circle to the area of the original square is *closest* in value to
   A. 4/5   B. 3/5   C. 2/3   D. 1/2

   7._____

8. A pound of water is evaporated from 6 pounds of sea water containing 4% salt. The percentage of salt in the *remaining* solution is
   A. 3 1/3   B. 4   C. 4 4/5   D. none of these

   8._____

9. If a cubic inch of a metal weighs 2 pounds, a cubic foot of the *same* metal weighs
   A. 8 pounds   B. 24 pounds   C. 288 pounds   D. none of these

   9._____

10. Assume that, according to the Federal income tax law, if the taxable income in the case of a separate return is over $4,000, but not over $6,000, the tax is $840 + 26% of the excess over $4,000.
If a taxpayer files a separate tax return and his taxable income is $5,500, the tax is

   A. $690   B. $1,230   C. $1,370   D. none of these

3 (#3)

SOLUTIONS TO ARITHMETICAL REASONING

1. Answer: (C) 48 miles per hour
   120 miles = 2 hours (60 mph)
   120 miles = 3 hours (40 mph)
   240 miles = 5 hours = average of 48 mph

2. Answer: (C) 3 inches
   Change 2 1/2 to 20/8   Change 1 7/8 to 15/8
   Ratio is 20 to 15 or 4 to 3.
   If the longer dimension is 4 inches, then the shorter is 3 inches.

3. Answer: (B) 1,024 feet
   s = 16 × 8² or 16 × 64 or 1024 feet

4. Answer: (A) $(75)^{10}$
   Because the 75 is constant, one needs only to add the exponents (7 and 3). Therefore, the product is 75^{10}.

5. Answer: (C) 80 miles
   6 ÷ 3/4 = 6 × 4/3 = 24/3 or 8
   8 × 10 miles = 80 miles

6. Answer: (A) increases in value
   By increasing the value of my (by substituting numbers for letters), it is obvious that d increases in value.

7. Answer: (A) 4/5
   Area of square = 36 square inches
   Area of circle = π^2
   = π 9 (3 × 3)
   = 3 1/7 × 9
   = 28 2/7

   $$\frac{28\ 2/7}{36} = \frac{198}{7} \times \frac{1}{36} = \frac{198}{252}$$

   ```
           .78 = 78%
   252)198.00
        176 4
         21 60
         20 16
          1 44
   ```

   78% is closest to 4/5 (80%)

8. Answer: (C) 4 4/5
.04 × 6 = .24 lbs. of salt in 6 lbs. of salt water
When a pound of water is evaporated, the salt content remains the same.

```
      .24
   5).24
      .04   4/5 = 4 4/5%
```

9. Answer: (D) none of these
1728 cubic inches = 1 cubic foot
1 cubic inch   = 2 pounds
1728 cubic inches = 3,456 pounds

10. Answer: (B) $1,230

$5,500
-4,000
$1,500 (excess over 4000)

$1500 × 25% = $390.00
              +840.00
              $1230.00 (tax)

TEST 4

DIRECTIONS: Each question or incomplete statement is followed by several suggested answers or completions. Select the one that BEST answers the question or completes the statement. *PRINT THE LETTER OF THE CORRECT ANSWER IN THE SPACE AT THE RIGHT.*

1. If the number of square inches in the area of a circle is equal to the number of inches in its circumference, the DIAMETER of the circle is 1.____
    A. 4 inches B. 3 inches C. 1 inch D. none of these

2. The *least common multiple* of 20, 24, 32 is 2.____
    A. 900 B. 1,920 C. 15,360 D. none of these

3. Six quarts of a 20% solution of alcohol in water are mixed with 4 quarts of a 60% solution of alcohol in water. The *alcoholic* strength of the mixture is 3.____
    A. 80% B. 50% C. 36% D. none of these

4. To find the radius of a circle whose circumference is 60 inches, 4.____
    A. multiply 60 by π
    B. divide 60 by 2π
    C. divide 30 by 2π
    D. divide 60 by π and extract the square root of the result

5. A micromillimeter is defined as one millionth of a millimeter. A length of 17 micromillimeters may be represented by 5.____
    A. .00017 mm. B. 0000017 mm.
    C. .000017 mm. D. .00000017 mm.

6. If 9x + 5 = 23, the numerical value of 18x + 5 is 6.____
    A. 46 B. 41 C. 32 D. 23 + 9x

7. When the fractions 2/3, 5/7, 8/11 and 9/13 are arranged in ascending order of size, the result is 7.____
    A. 8/11, 5/7, 9/13, 2/3 B. 5/7, 8/11, 2/3, 9/13
    C. 2/3, 8/11, 5/7, 9/13 D. 2/3, 9/13, 5/7, 8/11

8. If the outer diameter of a metal pipe is 2.84 inches and the inner diameter is 1.94 inches, the *thickness* of the metal is 8.____
    A. .45 of an inch B. .90 of an inch C. 1.94 inches D. 2.39 inches

9. An office manager employs 3 typists at $450 per week, 2 general clerks at $400 per week, and a messenger at $320 per week. The *average* weekly wage of these part-time employees is 9.____
    A. $372.50 B. $390.00 C. $411.70 D. none of these

10. A rectangular bin 4 feet long, 3 feet wide, and 2 feet high is solidly packed with bricks whose dimensions are 8 inches, 4 inches, and 2 inches. The *number* of bricks in the bin is 10.____
    A. 54 B. 648 C. 1,298 D. none of these

SOLUTIONS TO ARITHMETICAL REASONING

1. Answer: (A) 4 inches
   Assume there are 100 square inches in the area of a circle and 100 inches in its circumference.
   A = 1/2Cr
   100 = 1/2 × Xr
   50r = 100
   r = 2
   d = 4

2. Answer: (D) none of these
   2)20 – 24 - 32
   2)10 – 12 – 16
   2)20 – 24 – 32
      5 – 3 – 4

   2 × 2 × 2 × 5 × 3 × 4 = 480

3. Answer: (C) 36%
   6 quarts × 20% = 120%
   4 quarts × 60% = 240%
   10 quarts = 360%
   1 quart = 36%

4. Answer: (B) divide 60 by 2

   C = 2r

   2πr = 60

   2r = 60/π

   r = (60/π) × (1/2)

   r = 60/(2π)

5. Answer: (C) .000017 mm.
   1 micromillimeter = .000001 mm.
   17 micromillimeters = .000017 mm.

6. Answer: (B) 41
   9x + 5 = 23
   9x = 23 – 5 or 9x = 18
   x = 2
   18x + 5 = 36 + 5 or 41

7. Answer: (D) 2/3, 9/13, 5/7, 8/11
   Find the least common denominator = 3003

   2/3 = 2002/3003, 9/13 = 2079/3003,   5/7 = 2145/3003, 8/11 = 2184/3003
   Correct order is 2/3, 9/13, 5/7, 8/11

3 (#4)

8. Answer: (A) .45 of an inch

2.84 inches	=	outer diameter
1.94 inches	=	inner diameter
.90 inches	=	thickness (both sides)
.45 inches	=	thickness (one side)

9. Answer: (C) $41.17

   3 × 45 = $135
   2 × 40 = 80

   $\frac{1}{6} \times 32 = \frac{32}{\$247}$

   $247 ÷ 6 = $41 1/6 or $41.17

10. Answer: (B) 648

    There are 1728 cu. inches in 1 cu. ft. (12 × 12 × 12)
    4 × 3 × 2 = 24 cu.ft. × 1728 = 41472 cu. in. ÷ 64 (8 × 4 × 2) = 648 bricks

TEST 5

DIRECTIONS: Each question or incomplete statement is followed by several suggested answers or completions. Select the one that BEST answers the question or completes the statement. *PRINT THE LETTER OF THE CORRECT ANSWER IN THE SPACE AT THE RIGHT.*

1. If x is less than 10, and y is less than 5, it follows that 1.____
   A. x is greater than y
   B. x = 2y
   C. x-y = 5
   D. x+y is less than 15

2. A dealer sells an article at a loss of 50% of the cost. Based on the selling price, the *loss* is 2.____
   A. 25%
   B. 50%
   C. 100%
   D. none of these

3. If 8 men get together at a reunion and each man shakes hands once with each of the others, the *total number* of handshakes is 3.____
   A. 49
   B. 56
   C. 64
   D. 28

4. The world record for cycling a stretch of 20 kilometers is 26 minutes. This corresponds to an average speed of, *approximately*, 4.____
   A. 29 miles per hour
   B. 46 miles per hour
   C. 32 miles per hour
   D. none of these

5. The sum, s, of n consecutive integers beginning with 1 can be found by use of the formula $s = \frac{n(n+1)}{2}$. The sum of the *first 100 consecutive integers* is 5.____
   A. 5,001
   B. 5,050
   C. 10,000
   D. 10,100

6. Of the following, the value of $\frac{\sqrt[3]{64.32}}{\sqrt{.041}}$ is closest to 6.____
   A. 400
   B. 200
   C. 20
   D. 16

7. If each edge of a cube is increased by 2 inches, the 7.____
   A. volume is increased by 8 cubic inches
   B. area of each face is increased by 4 square inches
   C. diagonal of each face is increased by 2 inches
   D. sum of the edges is increased by 24 inches

8. In a school in which 40% of the enrolled students are boys, 80% of the boys are present on a certain day. If 1,152 boys are present, the total school enrollment is 8.____
   A. 1,440
   B. 2,880
   C. 3,600
   D. none of these

2 (#5)

9. An agent received a commission of d% of the selling price of a house. If the commission amounted to $600, the selling price, in dollars, was

   A. $\dfrac{60,000}{d}$ B. 600/d   C. 6d   D. 600d

9.____

10. A ship sails due north from a position 5 28' South Latitude to a position 6 43' North Latitude. Given that one minute of latitude is equivalent to 1 nautical mile, the ship has sailed a distance of _____ nautical miles
   A. 75   B. 371   C. 731   D. 1,211

10.____

3 (#5)

SOLUTIONS TO ARITHMETICAL REASONING

1. Answer: (D) x + y is less than 15
   If x is less than 10 and y is less than 5, then x + y MUST be less than 15. None of the others is possible.

2. Answer: (C) 100%
   Based on selling price, the formula is written:
   Cost − Loss = Selling Price
   100% - 50% = 50%
   Loss = 100% of the Selling Price (loss equal to Selling Price)

3. Answer: (D) 28
   A shakes hands with the other 7
   B shakes hands with the other 6 (has already shaken A's)
   and so on……. Thus 7, 6, 5, 4, 3, 2, 1 = 28 handshakes

4. Answer: (A) 29 miles per hour
   1 kilometer = 5/8 of a mile
   20 kilometers = 20 × 5/8 = 12 1/2 miles
   12 1/2 miles : 26 minutes = x : 60 minutes
   26x = 750
   x = 28+ or 29 miles per hour

5. Answer: (B) 5,050

   $s = \dfrac{n(n+1)}{2}$ $s = \dfrac{100(100+1)}{2}$ $s = \dfrac{10,100}{2}$ $s = 5,050$

6. Answer: (C) 2

   $\sqrt[3]{64.32} = 4.01$ $\dfrac{4}{.2} = 4 \times \dfrac{10}{2} = 20$

   $\sqrt{.041} - .202$

7. Answer: (D) the sum of the edges is increased by 24 inches. Since there are 12 edges to a cube and each edge is increased by 2 inches, the total increase is 24 inches.

8. Answer: (C) 3,600

   $1152 \div \dfrac{8}{10} = 1440 = 1440$ boys enrolled (1152 × 10/8)

   $1440 \div \dfrac{4}{10} = 1440 \times \dfrac{10}{4}$ (total school enrollment)

9. Answer: (A) $\dfrac{60,000}{d}$

4 (#5)

$600 \div d = 600 \times \dfrac{100}{d} = \dfrac{60,000}{d}$

10. Answer: (C) 731 nautical miles

```
   5° 28'                    1° = 60'
   6° 43'                   11° = 660'
  11° 71'                      +  71'
                                731'
```

1' = 1 nautical mile
731' = 731 nautical miles

QUANTITATIVE COMPARISON COMMENTARY

The item-type designated as *QUANTITATIVE COMPARISON* is a novel form of mathematics problem stressing the finest and highest types of conceptualizing, reasoning, and evaluating.

The examinee is directed to compare two quantities and to decide, on the basis of the information given, which, if either, is greater.

For example, if you were requested to compare 5/8 X 1/4 X 1/5 X 1/6 with 3/7 X 1/4 X 1/5 X 1/6, it would NOT be necessary to compute *each* product. It would suffice, *preferably,* to see at once that 1/4 X 1/5 X 1/6 is common to both items and, immediately, to appreciate that 5/8 > 3/7. Therefore, 5/8 X 1/4 X 1/5 X 1/6 must be, of course, the greater quantity.

Fundamental to the quantitative-comparison question are the concepts *greater than, less than,* and *equal to,* and the meaning and use of the symbols, > ("greater than"), and < ("less than"), which should be overlearned since these symbols appear or are implied in practically every question.

It would be wise to review the basic principles and concepts of algebra and geometry as a necessary preparation for this question-type. However, the candidate is advised that advanced mathematics is *not* required in the solution or interpretation of any of these problems.

Following are the directions in detail for the quantitative-comparison question:

DIRECTIONS: Each question in this section consists of two quantities, one in Column A and one in Column B. You are to compare the two quantities and, on the answer sheet, blacken space
- (A) if the quantity in Column A is the greater;
- (B) if the quantity in Column B is the greater;
- (C) if the two quantities are equal;
- (D) if the relationship cannot be determined from the information given.

<u>DIAGRAMS</u>

Position of points, angles, regions, etc., can be assumed to be in the order shown.

Figures are NOT NECESSARILY drawn to scale and may NOT agree to measure shown unless a note states that the figure is drawn to scale,
   Lines shown as straight can be assumed to be straight.
   Figures are assumed to lie in the plane unless otherwise indicated,

Note: All numbers used are real numbers, In a question, information concerning one or both of the quantities to be compared is centered above the two columns, A symbol that appears in both columns represents the same thing in Column A as it does in Column B.

Definitions of symbols:

    < is less than   ≤ is less than or equal to

    > is greater than   ≥ is greater than or equal to

    ⊥ is perpendicular to   ∥ is parallel to

                                    ≠ is not equal to

SAMPLE QUESTIONS

DIRECTIONS: See page 1.

1.   <u>Column A</u>   <u>Column B</u>   1._____
               2 X 6   2 + 6

The correct answer is A, since, obviously, 2 *times* a number is patently greater than 2 *more than* that same number.

Questions 2-4.

DIRECTIONS: Questions 2-4 refer to △ PQR.

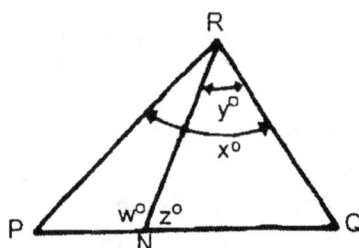

2.   Column A   Column B   2._____
                  PN   NQ

The correct answer is D, since nothing can be assumed about measures from the figure.

3.   Column A   Column B   3._____
                  Y   X

The correct answer is B, since N is between P and Q.

4.   Column A   Column B   4._____
                w + z   180

The correct answer is C, since PQ is a straight line.

EXAMINATION SECTION
TEST 1

DIRECTIONS: Each question in this section consists of two quantities, one in Column A and one in Column B. You are to compare the two quantities and, on the answer sheet, blacken space
    (A) if the quantity in Column A is the greater;
    (B) if the quantity in Column B is the greater;
    (C) if the two quantities are equal;
    (D) if the relationship cannot be determined from the information given.

1. Column A   Column B

$BA \perp AD$
$x° = y°$
$AE \perp BD$

BE   ED

2. Column A   Column B

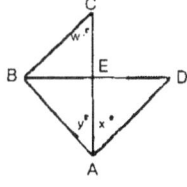

$BA \perp BC$
$BA = BC$
$AC \perp BD$

W°   X°

3. Column A   Column B

$e \perp d$
$e \perp b$
$a \parallel c$

a   c

4. Column A   Column B

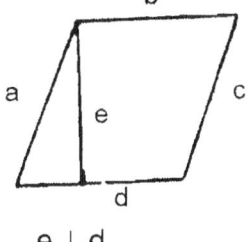

$e \perp d$
$e \perp$

b   d

143

2 (#1)

5. **Column A**   **Column B**   5.____

$$a \times b \geq c \times d$$
$$a > d$$

b   c

6. **Column A**   **Column B**   6.____

$a > b < c$ $a > 0$
$a < c$ $b > 0$
     $c > 0$

c − b   c − a

7. **Column A**   **Column B**   7.____

$$a \leq 0$$

a^2 a − a

8. **Column A**   **Column B**   8.____

$$\sqrt{x^2 + 16} = x + 4$$

x   zero

9. **Column A**   **Column B**   9.____

Given: Steel melts at 2800° F at the constant rate of 1 cubic inch per half hour

Time needed to melt a solid rectangular steel object, 1 foot wide, 2 feet high, 6 inches deep   One month

10. **Column A**   **Column B**   10.____

Circle has center P

(figure: circle with center P, diameter 8", point X on circle, XZ = 6, angle at P = 9°, Z on circle)

Area of given circle $\sqrt{2500}$ sq. in.

KEY (CORRECT ANSWERS)

1. C
2. D
3. C
4. D
5. D

6. A
7. D
8. C
9. A
10. A

TEST 2

DIRECTIONS: Each question in this section consists of two quantities, one in Column A and one in Column B. You are to compare the two quantities and, on the answer sheet, blacken space
- (A) if the quantity in Column A is the greater;
- (B) if the quantity in Column B is the greater;
- (C) if the two quantities are equal;
- (D) if the relationship cannot be determined from the information given.

Questions 1-2.

DIRECTIONS: Questions 1-2 are based upon the description given below.

A line is drawn from P (center of given circle) to X (point outside circle). Another line is drawn from P to Z (a point on the circle). Another line connects X and Z and is tangent to the circle at A.

1. Column A
   Line PZ
   Column B
   Line PX
   1.____

2. Column A
   Angle a°
   Column B
   Angle b°
   2.____

3. Column A
   7/2
   Column B
   $\sqrt{10}$
   3.____

4. Column A
   Number of one-inch links-in a 12-foot chain
   Column B
   Number of one-foot links in a 45-yard chain
   4.____

5. Column A
   The number of sides in a pentagon
   Column B
   The cube root of 343 minus the cube root of 27
   5.____

6. Column A
   9/16 x 4/3 x 3 x 1/2 x 8
   Column B
   8/16 x 3/4 x 11 x 4 x 5/8
   6.____

7. Column A | Column B | 7._____

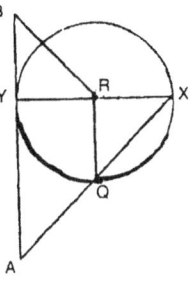

AY‖QR

QR ⊥ YX

BR>AQ

AX | AB

8. Column A | Column B | 8._____

$3x=4y$
$4x=x^2+4$

7x | 9y+1

Questions 9-10.

DIRECTIONS: Questions 9-10 are based on the diagram of a circle appearing below.

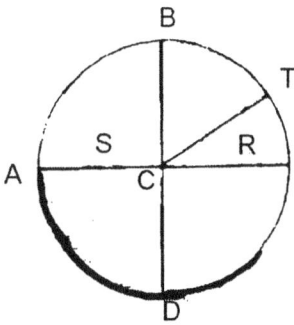

9. Column A | Column B | 9._____
Area ABC | Area ADC

10. Column A | Column B | 10._____
AC | CT

KEY (CORRECT ANSWERS)

1. B
2. B
3. A
4. A
5. A

6. B
7. D
8. B
9. D
10. D

TEST 3

DIRECTIONS: Each question in this section consists of two quantities, one in Column A and one in Column B. You are to compare the two quantities and, on the answer sheet, blacken space

    (A) if the quantity in Column A is the greater;
    (B) if the quantity in Column B is the greater;
    (C) if the two quantities are equal;
    (D) if the relationship cannot be determined from the information given.

1. | Column A | Column B |
|---|---|
| | CE∥FH |
| | GF=GB=FB |
| ∡CDG | 1/2 of ∡BOH |

2. | Column A | | Column B |
|---|---|---|
| ∡ADC + ∡FGB | CE∥FH | The total of all angles of a right triangle |

3. Column A   Column B

CE∥FH

∡FGB   ∡ADE

4. | Column A | Column B |
|---|---|
| | a ≤ 0 |
| | b ≤ 0 |
| | a ≠ b |
| b−a | b+a |

5. | Column A | Column B |
|---|---|
| 9 X 8 X 283 | 283 X 6 X 12 |

149

6. Column A — The average number of leaves shed per day by tree X during November if tree X shed all 300 of its leaves that month

   Column B — 10

7. Column A

   $a^3 + 1$

   $0 > a$

   Column B — 0

8. Column A

   $a - b$

   $a < 0$
   $b < 0$

   Column B — $a + b$

9. Column A

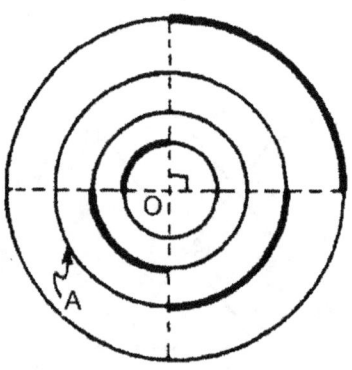

   All circles have center O.
   The diameter of the largest circle is 2d and the diameter of each other circle is 1/2 the diameter of the next larger circle.

   Total length of darkened areas

   Column B — Circumference of Circle A

10. Column A

    x

    $2x \frac{<x-4}{2}$

    Column B — x^3

KEY (CORRECT ANSWERS)

1. C
2. C
3. C
4. D
5. C

6. B
7. D
8. B
9. B
10. A

TEST 4

DIRECTIONS: Each question in this section consists of two quantities, one in Column A and one in Column B. You are to compare the two quantities and, on the answer sheet, blacken space
    (A) if the quantity in Column A is the greater;
    (B) if the quantity in Column B is the greater;
    (C) if the two quantities are equal;
    (D) if the relationship cannot be determined from the information given.

Questions 1-3.

DIRECTIONS: Questions 1-3 refer to the diagram below.

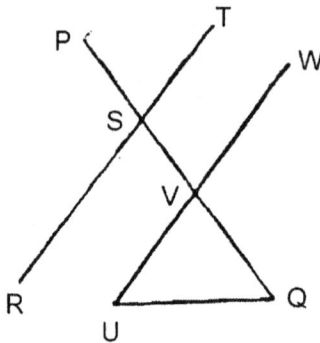

1.   Column A   RT ∥ UW   Column B   1.____
     ∡ UVQ   ∡ PST

2.   Column A   Column B   2.____
                          RT ∥ UW
   ∡FSR + ∡UVQ   180°

3.   Column A   Column B   3.____
                          RT ∥ UW

                       UV = VQ = UQ
   ∡ RSV   1/2 of ∡WVQ

4.   Column A.   Column B   4.____
     5/2
     5/2 $\sqrt{6}$

Questions 5-7.

2 (#4)

DIRECTIONS: Questions 5-7 refer to the diagram below:

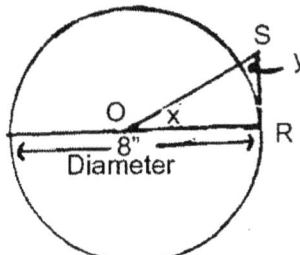

	Column A	Column B	
5.	Area of circle	500 sq. in.	5.___
6.	OR	OS	6.___
7.	∡X	∡Y	7.___
8.	a	a^3	8.___

$$2a < \frac{a}{2} - 2$$

Questions 9-10.

DIRECTIONS: Questions 9 and 10 refer to the diagram below:

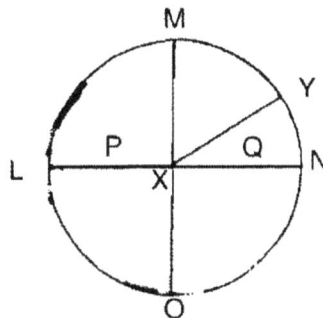

Point X bisects line LN
MO ⊥ LN

	Column A	Column B	
9.	Area LMX	Area LXO	9.___
10.	LX	XY	10.___

153

KEY (CORRECT ANSWERS)

1. C
2. C
3. C
4. A
5. A

6. B
7. D
8. A
9. D
10. D

EXAMINATION SECTION
TEST 1

DIRECTIONS: Each question or incomplete statement is followed by several suggested answers or completions. Select the one that BEST answers the question or completes the statement. *PRINT THE LETTER OF THE CORRECT ANSWER IN THE SPACE AT THE RIGHT.*

Questions 1-7.

DIRECTIONS: Questions 1 through 7 refer to the diagram that follows. Base your choice on the information given in the selection and on your own understanding of science.

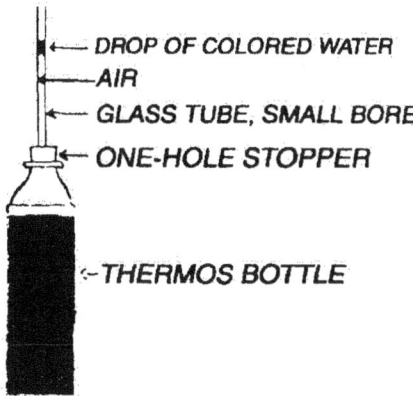

1. The device shown in the diagram above indicates changes that are measured MORE accurately by a(n)

    A. thermometer   B. hygrometer   C. anemometer
    D. hydrometer   E. barometer

1.____

2. If the device is placed in a cold refrigerator for 72 hours, which of the following is MOST likely to happen?

    A. The stopper will be forced out of the bottle.
    B. The drop of water will evaporate.
    C. the drop will move downward.
    D. The drop will move upward.
    E. No change will take place

2.____

3. When the device was carried in an elevator from the first floor to the sixth floor of a building, the drop of colored water moved about 1/4 inch in the tube. Which of the following is MOST probably true?

    A. The drop moved downward because there was a decrease in the air pressure.
    B. The drop moved upward because there was a decrease in the air pressure.
    C. The drop moved downward because there was an increase in the air temperature.
    D. The drop moved upward because there was an increase in the air temperature.
    E. The drop moved downward because there was an increase in the temperature and a decrease in the pressure.

3.____

4. The part of a thermos bottle into which liquids are poured consists of

   A. a single-walled, metal flask coated with silver
   B. two flasks, one of glass and one of silvered metal
   C. two silvered-glass flasks separated by a vacuum
   D. two silver flasks separated by a vacuum
   E. a single-walled glass flask with a silver-colored coating

5. The thermos bottle is MOST similar in principle to

   A. the freezing unit in an electric refrigerator
   B. radiant heaters
   C. solar heating systems
   D. storm windows
   E. a thermostatically controlled heating system

6. In a plane flying at an altitude where the air pressure is only half the normal pressure at sea level, the plane's altimeter should read APPROXIMATELY

   A. 3,000 feet   B. 9,000 feet   C. 18,000 feet
   D. 27,000 feet E. 60,000 feet

7. Which of the following is the POOREST conductor of heat?

   A. Air under a pressure of 1.5 pounds per square inch
   B. Air under a pressure of 15 pounds per square inch
   C. Unsilvered glass
   D. Silvered glass
   E. Silver

Questions 8-17.

DIRECTIONS: Questions 8 through 17 refer to the passage that follows. Base your choice on the information given in the passage *and on your own understanding of the subject.*

The formed elements of the blood are the red corpuscles or erythrocytes, the white corpuscles or leucocytes, the blood platelets, and the so-called blood dust or hemoconiae. Together, these constitute 30-40 percent by volume of the whole blood, the remainder being taken up by the plasma. In man, there are normally 5,000,000 red cells per cubic millimeter of blood; the count is somewhat lower in women. Variations occur frequently, especially after exercise or a heavy meal, or at high altitudes. Except in camels, which have elliptical corpuscles, the shape of the mammalian corpuscle is that of a circular, nonnucleated, bi-concave disk. The average diameter usually given is 7.7 microns, a value obtained by examining dried preparations of blood and considered by Ponder to be too low. Ponder's own observations, made on red cells in the fresh state, show the human corpuscle to have an average diameter of 8.8 microns. When circulating in the blood vessels, the red cell does not maintain a fixed shape but changes its form constantly, especially in the small capillaries. The red blood corpuscles are continually undergoing destruction, new corpuscles being formed to replace them. The average life of red corpuscles has been estimated by various investigators to be between three and six weeks. Preceding destruction, changes in the composition of the cells are believed to occur which render them less resistant. In the process of destruction, the lipids of the membrane are dissolved and the hemoglobin which is liberated is the most important, though probably not the only source of bilirubin. The belief that the liver is the only site of red celldestruction is no longer generally held. The leucocytes, of which there are several forms, usually number 7000 and 9000 per cubic millimeter of blood. These increase in number in disease, particularly when there is bacterial infection.

8. Leukemia is a disease involving the 8.____

   A. red cells B. white cells C. plasma
   D. blood platelets E. blood dust

9. "The erythrocytes in the blood are increased in number after a heavy meal." The paragraph implies that this 9.____

   A. is true B. holds only for camels
   C. is not true D. may be true
   E. depends on the number of white cells

10. When blood is dried, the red cells 10.____

    A. contract B. remain the same size C. disintegrate
    D. expand E. become elliptical

11. Ponder is PROBABLY classified as a professional 11.____

    A. pharmacist B. physicist C. psychologist
    D. physiologist E. psychiatrist

12. The term *erythema* when applied to skin conditions signifies 12.____

    A. redness B. swelling C. irritation
    D. pain E. roughness

13. Lipids are insoluble in water and soluble in such solvents as ether, chloroform and benzene. It may be inferred that the membrane of red cells MOST closely resemble 13.____

    A. egg white B. sugar C. bone D. butter
    E. cotton fiber

14. Analysis of a sample of blood yields cell counts of 4,800,000 erythrocytes and 16,000 leucocytes per cubic millimeter. These data suggest that the patient from whom the blood was taken 14.____

    A. is anemic
    B. has been injuriously invaded by germs
    C. has been exposed to high-pressure air
    D. has a normal cell count
    E. has lost a great deal of blood

15. Bilirubin, a bile pigment, is 15.____

    A. an end product of several different reactions
    B. formed only in the liver
    C. formed from the remnants of the dell membranes of erythrocytes
    D. derived from hemoglobin exclusively
    E. a precursor of hemoglobin

16. Bancroft found that the blood count of the natives in the Peruvian Andes differed from that usually accepted as normal. The blood PROBABLY differed in respect to

    A. leucocytes   B. blood platelets   C. cell shapes
    D. erythrocytes   E. hemoconiae

17. Hemoglobin is probably NEVER found

    A. free in the blood stream   B. in the red cells
    C. in women's blood   D. in the blood after exercise
    E. in the leucocytes

Questions 18-27.

DIRECTIONS: Questions 18 through 27 refer to the passage that follows. Base your choice on the information given in the passage *and on your own understanding of the subject.*

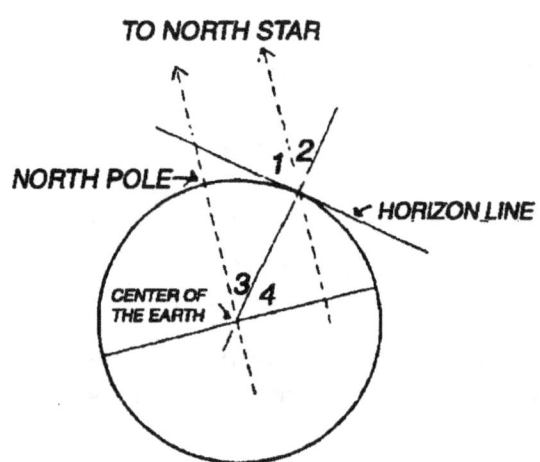

    The latitude of any point on the earth's surface is the angle between a plumb line dropped to the center of the earth from that point and the plane of the earth's equator. Since it is impossible to go to the center of the earth to measure latitude, the latitude of any point may be determined indirectly as shown in the accompanying diagram.
    It will be recalled that the axis of the earth, if extended outward, passes very near the North Star. Since the North Star is, for all practical purposes, infinitely distant, the line of sight to the North Star of an observer on the surface of the earth is virtually parallel with the earth's axis. Angle 1, then, in the diagram represents the angular distance of the North Star above the horizon. Angle 2 is equal to angle 3, because when two parallel lines are intersected by a straight line, the corresponding angles are equal. Angle 1 plus angle 2 is a right angle and so is angle 3 plus angle 4. Therefore, angle 1 equals angle 4 because when equals are subtracted from equals the results are equal.

18. If an observer finds that the angular distance of the North Star above the horizon is 30, his latitude is

    A. 15° N   B. 30° N   C. 60° N   D. 90° N   E. 120° N

19. To an observer on the equator, the North Star would be

    A. 30° above the horizon
    B. 60° above the horizon
    C. 90° above the horizon
    D. on the horizon
    E. below the horizon

20. To an observer on the Arctic Circle, the North Star would be

    A. directly overhead
    B. 23 1/2° above the horizon
    C. 66 1/2° above the horizon
    D. on the horizon
    E. below the horizon

21. The distance around the earth along a certain parallel of latitude is 3,600 miles. At this latitude, how many miles are there in one degree of longitude?

    A. 1 mile
    B. 10 miles
    C. 30 miles
    D. 69 miles
    E. 100 miles

22. At which of the following latitudes would the sun be directly overhead at noon on June 21?

    A. 0°   B. 23 1/2° S   C. 23 1/2° N   D. 66 1/2° N   E. 66 1/2° S

23. On March 21 the number of hours of daylight at places on the Arctic Circle is

    A. none   B. 8   C. 12   D. 16   E. 24

24. The distance from the equator to the 45th parallel, measured along a meridian, is APPROXIMATELY

    A. 450 miles
    B. 900 miles
    C. 1,250 miles
    D. 3,125 miles
    E. 6,250 miles

25. The difference in time between the meridians that pass through longitude 45°E and longitude 105°W is

    A. 6 hours
    B. 2 hours
    C. 8 hours
    D. 4 hours
    E. 10 hours

26. Which of the following is NOT a great circle or part of a great circle?

    A. Arctic Circle
    B. 100th meridian
    C. equator
    D. Shortest distance between New York and London
    E. Greenwich meridian

27. At which of the following places does the sun set earliest on June 21?

    A. Montreal, Canada
    B. Santiago, Chile
    C. Mexico City, Mexico
    D. Lima, Peru
    E. Manila, P.I.

28. At which of the following cities is the daily temperature range GREATEST?

    A. Key West
    B. Los Angeles
    C. Chicago
    D. New York City
    E. Denver

29. The MAXIMUM percentage of water vapor possible in the air is about

    A. 1%   B. 78%   C. .03%   D. 4%   E. 100%

30. When a mass of air rises, it is cooled CHIEFLY because

   A. it expands
   B. moisture condenses
   C. ice crystals are formed
   D. it mixes with cold air
   E. it is closer to cold outer space

31. An amateur pilot flying into a series of cold front thunderstorms should

   A. fly through without change of course
   B. fly around the thunderstorms
   C. land and get his plane into a hangar
   D. fly under the storm front
   E. fly over the top

32. Soaring pilots find MOST thermals

   A. about midmorning
   B. about 2 hours after noon
   C. in late afternoon
   D. Just after sunset
   E. in early morning

33. On a contour map, lines that are close together indicate that the land

   A. slopes gently B. is swampy C. slopes steeply
   D. is high E. is impassable

34. The planet that is NEAREST in size to the Earth is

   A. Mars   B. Venus   C. Mercury   D. Uranus   E. Jupiter

35. Of the total mass of the sun, planets, moons and other bodies in our solar system, the sun comprises APPROXIMATELY

   A. 1%   B. 10%   C. 50%   D. 90%   E. 99%

36. A sea cave at an altitude of 100 feet would indicate

   A. great tidal range B. severe storms
   C. uplift of land D. submergence of land
   E. rapid deposition of sediment

37. The element that makes up about 50% of the earth's crust is

   A. silicon B. nitrogen C. iron
   D. aluminum E. oxygen

38. Two elements obtained from the sea in commercial quantities are

   A. iron and sulfur B. nitrogen and argon
   C. copper and tin D. aluminum and iodine
   E. magnesium and bromine

39. Atoms of plutonium are composed of

   A. neutrons and protons
   B. electrons and neutrons
   C. electrons, neutrons and ions
   D. ions, protons and electrons
   E. neutrons, electrons and protons

40. Uranium used in making atomic bombs occurs in the mineral   40.____

    A. hematite   B. pitchblende   C. franklinite
    D. malachite   E. smithsonite

41. Which of the following is an explosive mixture?   41.____

    A. Oxygen and carbon monoxide
    B. Oxygen and caron dioxide
    C. Carbon dioxide and caron monoxide
    D. Carbon dioxide and hydrogen
    E. Nitrogen and carbon dioxide

42. Which of the following will react with baking soda to produce carbon dioxide?   42.____

    A. Table salt   B. Cane molasses   C. Granulated sugar
    D. Sweet cream   E. Wheat flour

43. Which of the following mechanisms requires NO external supply of oxygen?   43.____

    A. Diesel engines   B. Four-cycle gasoline engines
    C. Jet turbine engines   D. Rockets
    E. Two-cycle internal-combustion engines

44. In an operating radio tube the electrons flow from   44.____

    A. plate to grid   B. grid to plate
    C. plate to filament   D. filament to plate
    E. grid to filament

45. In hydroelectric stations, the energy of the turbines is applied directly to the operation of   45.____

    A. synchronous motors   B. water motors   C. steam engines
    D. generators   E. electric motors

46. A boy is given two similar bars of iron, which we shall call A and B. He finds that either   46.____
    end of A clings to either end of B, that either end of A clings to the middle of B and that
    neither end of B clings to the middle of A. He concludes CORRECTLY that

    A. both A and B are magnetized
    B. A is magnetized and B is not
    C. B is magnetized and A is not
    D. neither A nor B is magnetized
    E. B is magnetized over its entire length and A is not magnetized in the middle

47. Inductive reaoning is reasoning   47.____

    A. by analogy to similar situations
    B. from faulty premises
    C. after an event has taken place
    D. from a principle to a conclusion
    E. from observations to generalizations

48. If a coin is held 2 feet from an electric lamp, the shadow of the coin 6 feet from the lamp   48.____
    has an area that compares to the area of the coin as

    A. 12 to 1   B. 24 to 1   C. 3 to 1   D. 6 to 1   E. 9 to 1

49. The appliance cord for an electric flatiron is made of

   A. stranded copper wire covered with asbestos and rubber
   B. solid copper wire covered with asbestos and rubber
   C. rubber-covered stranded copper wire
   D. asbestos-covered nichrome wire
   E. rubber-covered nichrome wire

50. The distributor in an automobile engine controls the

   A. proportion of the electric current flowing to the lights and starter
   B. amount of electric current released from the storage battery
   C. flow of gasoline to the carburetor
   D. transmission of the spark occurrence to the spark plug
   E. amount of pressure on each brake drum

KEY (CORRECT ANSWERS)

1. A	11. D	21. B	31. C	41. A
2. C	12. A	22. C	32. C	42. D
3. B	13. D	23. C	33. C	43. D
4. C	14. B	24. D	34. B	44. D
5. D	15. A	25. E	35. E	45. D
6. C	16. D	26. A	36. C	46. B
7. A	17. E	27. B	37. E	47. E
8. B	18. B	28. E	38. E	48. E
9. D	19. D	29. D	39. E	49. A
10. A	20. C	30. A	40. B	50. D

TEST 2

DIRECTIONS: Each question or incomplete statement is followed by several suggested answers or completions. Select the one that BEST answers the question or completes the statement. *PRINT THE LETTER OF THE CORRECT ANSWER IN THE SPACE AT THE RIGHT.*

Questions 1-7.

DIRECTIONS: Questions 1 through 7 refer to the diagram that follows. Base your choice on the information given in the selection and on your own understanding of science.

1. The ignition coil in an automobile

   A. regulates the flow of current to the lights
   B. increases the voltage of the current to the spark plugs
   C. controls the charging rate of the battery
   D. boosts the voltage between the battery and the starting motor
   E. takes the place of the generator when the engine is not running

   1.____

2. When the gears of an automobile are shifted from "high" to "low," the

   A. power of the motor is increased
   B. force applied by the driving wheels is increased
   C. force applied by the motor is decreased
   D. speed of the driving wheels is increased
   E. transmission gears have increased the power

   2.____

3. If metal pipe is to be used to carry liquids or gases, the threaded portion is ALWAYS

   A. straight   B. tapered   C. fine   D. coarse   E. square

   3.____

4. Which of these fastening devices is a rivet?

   4.____

5. A substance mixed with cement and water to form the finishing coat on a concrete sidewalk is

   A. fill   B. sand   C. plaster of paris   D. mortar   E. gravel

   5.____

6. The board of fire underwriters requires inspection of

   A. house paint   B. roofing material
   C. furnace installation   D. hot-water pipes
   E. electric wiring

   6.____

7. Which tool is MOST generally used with a brace to bore a hole?

   A. Twist drill   B. Center drill   C. Countersink
   D. Auger bit   E. Rose reamer

   7.____

8. By what name is this tool commonly called?

   A. Nail set   B. Wedge   C. Pry bar   D. Cold chisel
   E. Gouge

9. Which is the MOST accurate instrument to use for marking on wood when laying out a joint in cabinet work?

   A. Knife   B. Pencil   C. Scriber   D. Brad awl   E. Nail

10. The fibers running lengthwise in a piece of cloth are called the

    A. heading   B. warp   C. weft   D. nap   E. pile

Questions 11-17.

DIRECTIONS: Questions 11 through 17 refer to the passage that follows. Base your choice on the information given in the selection *and on your own understanding of science*.

The higher forms of plants and animals, such as seed plants and vertebrates, are similar or alike in many respects but decidedly different in others. For example, both of these groups of organisms carry on digestion, respiration, reproduction, conduction, growth, and exhibit sensitivity to various stimuli. On the other hand, a number of basic differences are evident. Plants have no excretory systems comparable to those of animals. Plants have no heart or similar pumping organ. Plants are very limited in their movements. Plants have nothing similar to the animal nervous system. In addition, animals can not synthesize carbohydrates from inorganic substances. Animals do not have special regions of growth, comparable to terminal and lateral meristems in plants, which persist throughout the life span of the organism. And, finally, the animal cell "wall" is only a membrane, while plant cell walls are more rigid, usually thicker, and may be composed of such substances as cellulose, lignin, pectin, cutin, and suberin. These characteristics are important to an understanding of living organisms and their functions and should, consequently, be carefully considered in plant and animal studies.

11. Which of the following do animals lack?

    A. Ability to react to stimuli
    B. Ability to conduct substances from one place to another
    C. Reproduction by gametes
    D. A cell membrane
    E. A terminal growth region

12. Which of the following statements is FALSE?

    A. Animal cell "walls" are composed of cellulose.
    B. Plants grow as long as they live.
    C. Plants produce sperms and eggs.
    D. All vertebrates have hearts.
    E. Wood is dead at maturity.

13. Respiration in plants takes place 13._____

   A. only during the day
   B. only in the presence of carbon dioxide
   C. both day and night
   D. only at night
   E. only in the presence of certain stimuli

14. An example of a vertebrate is the 14._____

   A. earthworm   B. starfish   C. amoeba
   D. cow   E. insect

15. Which of the following statements is TRUE? 15._____

   A. All animals eat plants as a source of food.
   B. Respiration, in many ways, is the reverse of photosynthesis.
   C. Man is an invertebrate animal.
   D. Since plants have no hearts, they can not develop high pressure in their cells.
   E. Plants can not move.

16. Which of the following do plants lack? 16._____

   A. A means of movement   B. Pumping structures
   C. Special regions of growth   D. Reproduction by gametes
   E. A digestive process

17. A substance that can be synthesized by green plants but NOT by animals is 17._____

   A. protein   B. cellulose   C. carbon dioxide
   D. uric acid   E. water

Questions 18-27.

DIRECTIONS: Questions 18 through 27 refer to the passage that follows. Base your choice on the information given in the selection *and on your own understanding of the subject.*

The discovery of antitoxin and its specific antagonistic effect upon toxin furnished an opportunity for the accurate investigation of the relationship of a bacterial antigen and its antibody. Toxin-antitoxin reactions were the first immunological processes to which experimental precision could be applied, and the discovery of principles of great importance resulted from such studies. A great deal of the work was done with diphtheria toxin and antitoxin and the facts elucidated with these materials are in principle applicable to similar substances.

The simplest assumption to account for the manner in which an antitoxin renders a toxin innocuous would be that the antitoxin destroys the toxin. Roux and Buchner, however, advanced the opinion that the antitoxin did not act directly upon the toxin, but affected it indirectly through the mediation of tissue cells. Ehrlich, on the other hand, conceived the reaction of toxin and antitoxin as a direct union, analogous to the chemical neutralization of an acid by a base.

The conception of toxin destruction was conclusively refuted by the experiments of Calmette. This observer, working with snake poison, found that the poison itself (unlike most other toxins) possessed the property of resisting heat to 100 degrees C, while its specific antitoxin, like other antitoxins, was destroyed at or about 70 degrees C. Nontoxic mixtures of the two substances, when subjected to heat, regained their toxic properties. The natural inference from these observations was that the toxin in the original mixture had not been destroyed, but had been merely inactivated by the presence of the antitoxin and again set free after destruction of the antitoxin by heat.

18. Both toxins and antitoxins ordinarily

    A. are completely destroyed at body temperatures
    B. are extremely resistant to heat
    C. can exist only in combination
    D. are destroyed at 180° F
    E. are products of nonliving processes

19. Most toxins can be destroyed by

    A. bacterial action   B. salt solutions
    C. boiling   D. diphtheria antitoxin
    E. other toxins

20. Very few disease organisms release a true toxin into the blood stream. It would follow, then, that

    A. studies of snake venom reactions have no value
    B. studies of toxin-antitoxin reactions are of little importance
    C. the treatment of most diseases must depend upon information obtained from study of a few
    D. antitoxin plays an important part in the body defense against the great majority of germs
    E. only toxin producers are dangerous

21. A person becomes susceptible to infection again immediately after recovering from

    A. mumps   B. tetanus   C. diphtheria   D. smallpox
    E. tuberculosis

22. City people are more frequently immune to communicable diseases than country people are because

    A. country people eat better food
    B. city doctors are better than country doctors
    C. the air is more healthful in the country
    D. country people have fewer contacts with disease carriers
    E. there are more doctors in the city than in the country

23. The substance that provide us with immunity to disease are found in the body in the

    A. blood serum   B. gastric juice   C. urine
    D. white blood cells E. red blood cells

24. A person ill with diphtheria would MOST likely be treated with

    A. diphtheria toxin   B. diphtheria toxoid
    C. dead diphtheria germs   D. diphtheria antitoxin
    E. live diphtheria germs

25. To determine susceptibility to diphtheria, an individual may be given the   25.____

    A. Wassermann test   B. Schick test   C. Widal test
    D. Dick test   E. Kahn test

26. Since few babies under six months of age contract diphtheria, young babies PROBABLY   26.____

    A. are never exposed to diphtheria germs
    B. have high body temperatures that destroy the toxin if acquired
    C. acquire immunity from their mothers
    D. acquire immunity from their fathers
    E. are too young to become infected

27. Calmette's findings   27.____

    A. contradicted both Roux and Buchner's opinion and Ehrlich's conception
    B. contradicted Roux and Buchner, but supported Ehrlich
    C. contradicted Ehrlich, but supported Roux and Buchner
    D. were consistent with both theories
    E. had no bearing on the point at issue

Questions 28-37.

DIRECTIONS: Questions 28 through 37 refer to the passage that follows. Base your choice on the information given in the selection *and on your own understanding of the subject.*

Sodium chloride, being by far the largest constituent of the mineral matter of the blood, assumes special significance in the regulation of water exchanges in the organism. And, as Cannon has emphasized repeatedly, these latter are more extensive and more important than may at first thought appear. He points out "there are a number of circulations of the fluid out of the body and back again, without loss." Thus, for example, it is estimated that from a quart to a quart and one-half of water daily "leaves the body" when it enters the mouth as saliva; another one or two quarts are passed out as gastric juice; and perhaps the same amount is contained in the bile and the secretions of the pancreas and the intestinal wall. This large volume of water enters the digestive processes; and practically all of it reabsorbed through the intestinal wall, where it performs the equally important function of carrying in the digested foodstuffs. These and other instances of what Cannon calls "the conservative use of water in our bodies" involve essentially osmotic pressure relationships in which the concentration of sodium chloride plays an important part.

28. This passage implies that   28.____

    A. the contents of the alimentary canal are not to be considered within the body
    B. sodium chloride does not actually enter the body
    C. every particle of water ingested is used over and over again
    D. water can not be absorbed by the body unless it contains sodium chloride
    E. substances can pass through the intestinal wall in only one direction

29. According to this passage, which of the following processes requires MOST water? The

   A. absorption of digested foods
   B. secretion of gastric juice
   C. secretion of saliva
   D. production of bile
   E. concentration of sodium chloride solution

30. A body fluid that is NOT saline is

   A. blood
   B. urine
   C. bile
   D. gastric juice
   E. saliva

31. An organ that functions as a storage reservoir from which large quantities of water are reabsorbed into the body is the

   A. kidney
   B. liver
   C. large intestine
   D. mouth
   E. pancreas

32. Water is reabsorbed into the body by the process of

   A. secretion
   B. excretion
   C. digestion
   D. osmosis
   E. oxidation

33. Digested food enters the body PRINCIPALLY through the

   A. mouth
   B. liver
   C. villi
   D. pancreas
   E. stomach

34. The metallic element found in the blood in compound form and present there in larger quantities than any other metallic element is

   A. iron
   B. calcium
   C. magnesium
   D. chlorine
   E. sodium

35. An organ that removes water from the body and prevents its reabsorption for use in the body processes is the

   A. pancreas
   B. liver
   C. small intestine
   D. lungs
   E. large intestine

36. In which of the following processes is sodium chloride removed MOST rapidly from the body?

   A. Digestion
   B. Breathing
   C. Oxidation
   D. Respiration
   E. Perspiration

37. Which of the following liquids would pass from the alimentary canal into the blood MOST rapidly?

   A. A dilute solution of sodium chloride in water
   B. Gastric juice
   C. A concentrated solution of sodium chloride in water
   D. Digested food
   E. Distilled water

38. The reason why it is unsafe to drink ocean water even under conditions of extreme thirst is that it

   A. would reduce the salinity of the blood to a dangerous level
   B. contains dangerous disease germs
   C. contains poisonous salts

D. would greatly increase the salinity of the blood
E. would cause salt crystals to form in the blood stream

39. When air rises from the surface of the earth, it

    A. contracts and grows warmer
    B. contracts and grows cooler
    C. expands and grows warmer
    D. expands and grows cooler
    E. increases in density

40. The approach of a warm front is USUALLY attended by

    A. cumulus clouds and thunderstorms
    B. stratus clouds and moist air
    C. brisk, northwesterly winds
    D. a rising barometer
    E. clear, dry air

41. A type of air mass that originates in the United States is the

    A. polar continental
    B. polar Atlantic
    C. polar Pacific
    D. tropical gulf
    E. tropical continental

42. The prevailing winds in New York State are

    A. anticyclones
    B. westerlies
    C. trade winds
    D. easterlies
    E. cyclones

43. A meteorologist in New York State would NOT regard as important for weather prediction

    A. the type of clouds in the sky
    B. the weather in Canada, Mexico and Cuba
    C. a change of direction of the wind
    D. a change in the phase of the moon
    E. a change of temperature of the air

44. Which of the following would be of SLIGHT interest to present-day meteorologists?

    A. Winds
    B. Clouds
    C. Precipitation
    D. Fronts
    E. Meteors

45. A cyclonic condition is developing rapidly and is traveling north north-east accompanied by rains and rising temperature. Which of the following important factors was omitted from this report?

    A. Barometric tendency
    B. Precipitation
    C. Storm's path
    D. Temperature tendency
    E. Wind velocity

46. Granite is a rock that was made by

    A. the cementation of sediments
    B. fire in the depths of the earth
    C. the compression of sediments
    D. the cooling of lava deep beneath the earth's surface
    E. the cooling of lava from volcanoes

47. The rate of erosion of cultivated fields with moderate slope can be reduced by 47.____

    A. leaving the fields unplanted every other year
    B. planting such crops as corn and potatoes
    C. planting strips of grass up and down the slope
    D. plowing across the slope
    E. planting firm sod around the fields

48. The PRINCIPAL reason for adding agricultural lime to soils is to 48.____

    A. improve the texture of the soil
    B. help to preserve the supply of humus
    C. supply materials to stiffen the stems of plants
    D. decrease the acidity of the soil
    E. supply calcium to the growing plants

49. The three elements found MOST commonly in commercial fertilizers are 49.____

    A. calcium, phosphorus, iron   B. nitrogen, phosphorus, potassium
    C. phosphorus, nitrogen, sulfur   D. calcium, potassium, iron
    E. magnesium, iron, calcium

50. When carbohydrates decompose in the soil, the end products are 50.____

    A. nitrates and carbon dioxide   B. carbon dioxide and water
    C. nitrates and nitrites   D. carbon monoxide and hydrogen
    E. nitrates and water

KEY (CORRECT ANSWERS)

1. B	11. E	21. E	31. C	41. D
2. B	12. A	22. D	32. D	42. B
3. B	13. C	23. A	33. C	43. D
4. A	14. D	24. D	34. E	44. E
5. B	15. B	25. B	35. D	45. E
6. E	16. B	26. C	36. E	46. D
7. D	17. B	27. D	37. E	47. D
8. D	18. D	28. A	38. D	48. D
9. C	19. C	29. A	39. D	49. B
10. B	20. C	30. D	40. B	50. B

TEST 3

DIRECTIONS: Each question or incomplete statement is followed by several suggested answers or completions. Select the one that BEST answers the question or completes the statement. *PRINT THE LETTER OF THE CORRECT ANSWER IN THE SPACE AT THE RIGHT.*

Questions 1-7.

DIRECTIONS: Questions 1 through 7 refer to the diagram that follows. Base your choice on the information given in the selection and on your own understanding of science.

1. Which of the following is a common insecticide used by gardeners?

    A. Alcohol B. Phosphoric acid C. Wood ashes
    D. Rotenone E. Nitrate of soda

2. The fruit of plants such as the tomato, cucumber, cherry and bean develops from the

    A. receptacle and closely associated stem
    B. petals and closely associated sepals
    C. stem and closely associated parts
    D. ovary and closely associated parts
    E. stamen and closely associated parts

3. The part of the toadstool or mushroom plant that is seen growing above the ground is of PRIMARY use in

    A. reproduction B. transpiration C. food storage
    D. digestion E. photosynthesis

4. Mendel crossed purebred, tall pea plants with dwarf pea plants. The offspring were all tall plants. When he crossed these tall plants with each other, the resulting offsprings were

    A. all tall
    B. about three-fourths tall and one-fourth dwarf
    C. about half tall and half dwarf
    D. about one-fourth tall and three-fourths dwarf
    E. nearly all dwarf

5. A plant cell can BEST be considered a(n)

    A. surface B. volume C. rectangle D. circle E. area

6. The stage in its life cycle in which the clothes moth does MOST harm to woolens is the

    A. blastula B. egg C. larva D. pupa E. adult

7. Lights in chicken houses stimulate egg production by

    A. stimulating in the chickens certain glands that affect formation of egg shells
    B. keeping hens awake so they can lay more eggs
    C. causing hens to consume more food, which results in more eggs produced
    D. increasing the vitamin D content in the hens
    E. controlling the ionization of the air

8. Which of the diseases listed below is caused by animal organism?

    A. Rickets   B. Hay fever   C. Typhoid fever   D. Malaria
    E. Chickenpox

9. Which of the following is a communicable disease?

    A. Scurvy   B. Cancer   C. Goiter
    D. Rabies   E. Nephritis

10. Sulfa drugs are produced CHIEFLY

    A. from a common mold
    B. from glands obtained from animals
    C. by chemical synthesis
    D. by a common bacterium
    E. from the bark of a tree

11. The human body is composed MAINLY of

    A. nitrogen, phosphorus, calcium   B. potassium, nitrogen, oxygen
    C. calcium, iron, potassium   D. carbon, hydrogen, oxygen
    E. iron, calcium, hydrogen

12. The stomach normally contains

    A. some hydrochloric acid   B. some nitric acid
    C. some sulfuric acid   D. some bases but no acids
    E. neither acids nor bases

13. Many of the organic compounds containing nitrogen are called

    A. oils   B. sugars   C. fats   D. starches   E. proteins

14. Man's normal complement of teeth during adulthood is

    A. 24   B. 28   C. 32   D. 36   E. 40

15. Development of the first set of teeth is begun

    A. before birth   B. 12 months after birth
    C. 15 months after birth   D. at birth
    E. 6 months after birth

16. Bacteria enlarge the dentine canals by

    A. eating the walls
    B. allowing the entrance of saliva
    C. stopping the flow of the lymph
    D. movements up and down the canals
    E. producing compounds that attack the walls

17. An experiment was conducted to determine the effect on dental health of introducing a chemical into the drinking water. This chemical contained

    A. magnetium   B. iodine   C. fluorine
    D. calcium   E. iron

18. Rheumatism is sometimes attributed to an abscessed tooth. The abscess may cause the condition by   18._____

    A. allowing bacteria to enter the blood
    B. pressing on a nerve
    C. allowing the lymph to escape
    D. producing poisons, which are absorbed
    E. using nutrients that should go to other parts of the body

19. An enzyme in gastric juice which aids in digesting protein is   19._____

    A. ptyalin   B. trypsin   C. amylopsin   D. pepsin
    E. maltase

20. To help prevent scarlet fever from spreading from one member of a household to other members, it is MOST essential to   20._____

    A. get a trained nurse
    B. keep the room temperature at 72° F
    C. have attendants change outer clothing upon leaving the sickroom
    D. remove all unnecessary accessories from the sickroom
    E. keep the patient in a warm room with windows closed

21. Of the following possible effects of an automobile accident, the condition that requires MOST immediate treatment is   21._____

    A. spinal dislocation   B. shock
    C. concussion   D. tetanus
    E. arterial bleeding

22. When rags used by painters to wipe up linseed oil catch fire spontaneously, it is because   22._____

    A. paint oil gives off oxygen readily
    B. paint oil oxidizes
    C. the cloth reduces the oxygen in the paint oil
    D. the paint oil reduces the oxygen in the cloth
    E. paint oil and cloth unite chemically

23. Alum is added to water in many municipal water systems to   23._____

    A. reduce unwanted dissolved gases
    B. remove objectionable flavors
    C. kill harmful bacteria
    D. soften the water
    E. remove sediment

24. Soap aids in cleaning because its action on greases and oils is to   24._____

    A. reduce them   B. oxidize them   C. emulsify them
    D. dissolve them   E. precipitate them

25. When a candle burns, the CHIEF products are   25._____

    A. carbon dioxide and carbon monoxide
    B. carbon dioxide and nitrogen
    C. carbon monoxide and nitrogen

D. carbon monoxide and water
E. carbon dioxide and water

26. Iron is removed from its oxide ores by

    A. roasting the ore
    B. reducing the ore with carbon
    C. oxidizing the ore with a blast of air
    D. melting the ore, thus allowing the iron to escape
    E. making a slag to absorb the oxides of the iron

27. A mineral much used as a source of iron is

    A. galena   B. hematite   C. franklinite   D. chromite
    E. halite

28. A gas generally used in incandescent lamps to increase their operating efficiency is

    A. freon   B. oxygen   C. neon   D. argon   E. chlorine

29. The meter whose readings are used in determining the amount of the monthly household electric bill measures

    A. voltage   B. electrical energy   C. power
    D. amperage   E. electrical resistance

30. Most household appliances using electric motors are made to operate on

    A. 110-volt alternating current   B. 110-volt direct current
    C. 32-volt direct current   D. 6-volt direct current
    E. 1 1/2-volt direct current

31. A bimetallic thermostat operates because

    A. metals expand when heated
    B. different metals expand at different rates when heated
    C. two metals will conduct electric currents at different rates
    D. a voltage is produced between the junctions of the two metals when one junction is heated
    E. different metals appear on different levels in the electromotive series

32. A transformer is used to change

    A. alternating current to direct current
    B. the voltage of alternating current
    C. the voltage of direct current
    D. the frequency of alternating current
    E. direct current to alternating current

33. One material much used for permanent magnets is

    A. steel   B. soft iron   C. copper   D. zinc   E. carbon

34. The surfaces of a thermos bottle are silvered to

   A. reduce convection
   B. reduce radiation
   C. reduce conduction
   D. keep out ultraviolet rays
   E. make cleaning easier

35. A temperature of 25° C is NEAREST to which of the following temperatures?

   A. 20° F   B. 40° F   C. 60° F   D. 80° F   E. 100° F

36. Ice floats because

   A. water becomes denser as it cools
   B. it contains so much air
   C. water expands when it freezes
   D. fish could not live in ponds if the ice sank to the bottom
   E. water expands as it cools from 4° C to 0° C

37. If a person facing a high cliff hears his echo 5 seconds after he shouts, the distance between the person and the cliff is about

   A. 1/4 mile   B. 1/2 mile   C. 3/4 mile
   D. 1 mile   E. 1 1/4 miles

38. The horizontal stabilizers of a plane are necessary to

   A. make the plane dive and climb
   B. make the plane bank on a turn
   C. keep the tail from bobbing up and down
   D. enable the pilot to turn right or left
   E. keep the plane from weaving from side to side

39. A good quality lumber for outside woodwork is

   A. basswood   B. hard maple   C. yellow birch
   D. white pine E. red gumwood

40. Knots in lumber are caused by

   A. boring insects   B. branches   C. winter injury
   D. decay   E. unequal growth

41. On which of the following woods MUST a paste filler be used during the finishing process?

   A. Basswood   B. Maple   C. Oak   D. Redgum   E. Cedar

42. In what order should the dimension of boards be listed when ordering lumber from a mill?

   A. Length, width, thickness
   B. Thickness, width, length
   C. Length, thickness, width
   D. Width, length, thickness
   E. Width, thickness, length

43. The number of a wood screw indicates its

   A. number of threads per inch
   B. style of point
   C. length
   D. style of head
   E. diameter

44. Half-and-half solder is an alloy composed of

   A. lead and tin
   B. tin and copper
   C. tin and zinc
   D. lead and brass
   E. zinc and lead

45. The process used to make earthenware waterproof is known as

   A. glazing   B. finishing   C. molding   D. firing
   E. decorating

46. Molds for casting clay are made of

   A. plaster of paris   B. galvanized iron   C. tin
   D. wood   E. cardboard

47. A tool used to cut the thread in a nut is a

   A. tap   B. die   C. reamer   D. drill   E. bolt

48. To draw vertical lines in drafting, one should use

   A. a T square   B. a rule   C. a triangle
   D. two triangles   E. a T square and triangle

49. The pica is a unit of measurement in

   A. ceramics   B. printing   C. toolmaking
   D. photography   E. textile design

50. Of the following, the fiber that is MOST weakened by being wet is

   A. cotton   B. rayon   C. linen   D. silk   E. wool

KEY (CORRECT ANSWERS)

1. D	11. D	21. E	31. B	41. C
2. D	12. A	22. B	32. B	42. B
3. A	13. E	23. E	33. A	43. E
4. B	14. C	24. C	34. B	44. A
5. B	15. A	25. E	35. D	45. A
6. C	16. E	26. B	36. C	46. A
7. A	17. C	27. B	37. B	47. A
8. D	18. D	28. D	38. C	48. E
9. D	19. D	29. B	39. D	49. B
10. C	20. C	30. A	40. B	50. E

TEST 4

DIRECTIONS: Each question or incomplete statement is followed by several suggested answers or completions. Select the one that BEST answers the question or completes the statement. *PRINT THE LETTER OF THE CORRECT ANSWER IN THE SPACE AT THE RIGHT.*

Questions 1-7.

DIRECTIONS: Questions 1 through 7 refer to the diagram that follows. Base your choice on the information given in the selection and on your own understanding of science.

1. The revolving part of an automobile generator is the

    A. cam B. slipring C. armature
    D. coil E. brushes

2. A by-product of soap manufacture is

    A. acetone B. benzine C. fat D. glycerin E. lye

3. When a certain quantity of water is decomposed by electrolysis, 60 cubic centimeters of hydrogen are produced. The number of cubic centimeters of oxygen obtained is

    A. 20 B. 30 C. 60 D. 120 E. 180

4. Of the following, the BEST conductor of heat is

    A. asbestos B. brass C. copper D. glass E. iron

5. The temperature of the air falls during the night, PRINCIPALLY because the earth loses heat by

    A. conduction B. convection C. insolation D. radiation
    E. reflection

6. The relative humidity of the air when dew forms is

    A. 10% B. 25% C. 50% D. 75% E. 100%

7. The low-pressure areas that bring stormy weather to New York State USUALLY come from the

    A. east B. north C. south D. southeast E. west

8. An instrument used to determine latitude is the

    A. altimeter B. barometer C. isobar D. hydrometer
    E. sextant

9. The earth rotates 30 degrees in

    A. 1 hour B. 2 hours C. 3 hours D. 4 hours E. 5 hours

10. The earth is NEAREST the sun in the month of

    A. January B. March C. June D. September E. December

11. All parts of the earth have 12 hours of daylight on

   A. December 21st B. June 21st C. July 21st
   D. March 21st E. November 21st

12. Eastern Double Daylight Saving Time corresponds to the standard time at the meridian of west longitude numbered

   A. 60 B. 75 C. 90 D. 105 E. 120

13. We see one-half of the lighted portion of the moon at the

   A. first quarter B. full moon C. new crescent
   D. new moon E. old crescent

14. A planet whose orbit is between the sun and the orbit of the earth is

   A. Jupiter B. Mars C. Pluto D. Saturn E. Venus

15. The changing position of the stars during the night is MAINLY the result of the

   A. inclination of the earth's axis
   B. rotation of the earth
   C. rotation of the stars
   D. revolution of the earth
   E. revolution of the stars

16. The gravational force of the moon is exerted

   A. only upon the side of the earth nearest the moon
   B. only upon the point on the earth nearest the moon
   C. upon the center of the earth only
   D. upon the entire earth
   E. upon the water surfaces of the earth but not upon the land surfaces

17. The work done by tides is gradually slowing down the earth's period of rotation. It is, therefore, reasonable to predict that, millions of years from now,

   A. the earth will be farther away from the moon than now
   B. the frequency of tides will be greater than now
   C. days will be shorter than they are now
   D. phases of the moon will change more rapidly than now
   E. lunar months will be longer than they are now

18. The earth's gravitational attraction is GREATEST at

   A. the North Pole
   B. the equator
   C. a point on the earth's surface directly under the moon
   D. a point on the earth's surface exactly opposite the moon
   E. a point 10 miles above the earth's surface, whatever the position of the moon

19. The part of the seed that develops into the young plant is called the

   A. cotyledon B. embryo C. hilum
   D. micropyle E. testa

20. The union of the sperm and the egg cells of flowers is called

   A. fertilization B. maturation C. parthenogenesis
   D. pollination E. sporulation

21. An insect that eats no food during the adult stage is the

   A. grasshopper B. bumblebee C. cricket
   D. Japanese beetle E. Cecropia moth

22. The image of an object is formed in the eye on the

   A. cornea B. pupil C. iris D. lens E. retina

23. An organ located above the diaphragm is the

   A. stomach B. liver C. heart D. pancreas E. spleen

24. Of the following, an organ that is NOT connected with the alimentary canal is the

   A. pancreas B. liver C. kidney D. salivary glands
   E. appendix

25. The ptyalin in saliva is a(n)

   A. auxin B. chalone C. enzyme D. hormone E. vitamin

26. Glucose is stored in the liver and muscles in the form of

   A. glycogen B. levulose C. glycocoll D. fat E. dextrose

27. A substance that is readily absorbed through the walls of the stomach is

   A. starch B. sugar C. alcohol D. amino acids
   E. ascorbic acid

28. The poisonouc character of carbon monoxide is due to its tendency to unite chemically with

   A. water B. synovial fluid C. cerebrospinal fluid
   D. hemoglobin E. gastric juice

29. A nutrient that contains nitrogen is

   A. fat B. protein C. starch D. sugar E. water

30. A substance that is a carbohydrate is

   A. glutenin B. stearin C. palmitin
   D. gliadin E. dextrin

31. A food that contains no vitamins is

   A. white potato B. cane sugar C. dried beans
   D. lard E. white bread

32. Of the following, the vegetable that contains the HIGHEST percentage of protein is the

   A. tomato B. cabbage C. carrot
   D. lima bean E. head lettuce

33. When bread is toasted, much of the starch is changed to

   A. dextrose   B. maltose   C. maltase   D. dextrin   E. biotin

34. A preparation of dead or weakened bacilli used for developing immunity to a disease is called a(n)

   A. vaccine   B. virus   C. culture medium   D. antitoxin
   E. immune serum

35. A disease caused by a virus is

   A. anthrax   B. dysentery   C. scurvy   D. smallpox
   E. tuberculosis

36. Of the following diseases, the one that is NOT caused by a filtrable virus is

   A. syphilis   B. yellow fever   C. measles   D. mumps
   E. infantile paralysis

37. A disease that may be prevented by the use of a vaccine is

   A. tuberculosis   B. poliomyelitis   C. rabies
   D. gonorrhea   E. dementia praecox

38. Immunity to diphtheria may be detected by the use of

   A. the Dick test   B. the Schick test
   C. arsphenamine   D. acetylsalicylate
   E. the Wassermann test

39. A substance used to treat malaria is

   A. sodium perborate   B. atabrine   C. penicillin
   D. salol   E. sulfathiazole

40. Silicosis may result from prolonged exposure to

   A. radium   B. poisonous gases   C. ragweed pollen
   D. metallic dusts   E. rock dusts

41. Trichinosis is a disease contracted MOSTLY from

   A. chicken   B. beef   C. pork   D. lamb   E. fish

42. Delay in the removal of an inflamed appendix sometimes results in

   A. peritonitis   B. gingivitis   C. gastritis
   D. phlebitis   E. meningitis

43. Blowing the nose hard during a cold is dangerous, PRIMARILY because the

   A. back pressure may force bacteria into the eustachian tubes
   B. lining of the nose may be damaged
   C. lungs may be overworked
   D. flow of mucus may be stopped
   E. nasal sinuses may burst

44. Mouth washes 44._____
    A. kill whatever germs are present in the mouth
    B. are effective in preventing diseases
    C. prevent germs from entering the mouth
    D. prevent the growth of germs in the mouth
    E. are of little or no health value

45. Dissolved impurities can be separated from water by 45._____
    A. aeration   B. chlorination   C. distillation
    D. filtration   E. settling

46. Lake or river water may be made safe to drink by letting the water stand one-half hour after adding 46._____
    A. two drops of tincture of iodine per quart
    B. one pint of ethyl alcohol per gallon
    C. one drop of sulfuric acid per quart
    D. 10 grams of table salt per gallon
    E. one aspirin tablet per pint

47. A dermatologist is a physician who specializes in the care of 47._____
    A. children   B. the hair   C. the skin   D. old people
    E. chronic diseases

48. Schizophrenia is a 48._____
    A. dangerous drug
    B. mental disorder
    C. dye used in staining tissue cells
    D. communicable disease
    E. hormone

49. An example of rationalization is 49._____
    A. building up an exaggerated tendency that is opposite to the unconscious wish
    B. justifying failure by means of arguments that excuse it
    C. complete forgetting of unfavorable experiences
    D. identifying oneself with a hero of some sort
    E. gratifying wishes by assuming an illness

50. The nutrient provided by milk and milk products that is MOST difficult to obtain from other common foods is 50._____
    A. vitamin A   B. calcium   C. complete protein
    D. niacin   E. vitamin C

KEY (CORRECT ANSWERS)

1. C	11. D	21. E	31. B	41. C
2. D	12. A	22. E	32. D	42. A
3. B	13. A	23. C	33. D	43. A
4. C	14. E	24. C	34. A	44. E
5. D	15. B	25. C	35. D	45. C
6. E	16. D	26. A	36. A	46. A
7. E	17. A	27. C	37. C	47. C
8. E	18. A	28. D	38. B	48. B
9. B	19. B	29. B	39. B	49. B
10. A	20. A	30. E	40. E	50. B

TEST 5

DIRECTIONS: Each question or incomplete statement is followed by several suggested answers or completions. Select the one that BEST answers the question or completes the statement. *PRINT THE LETTER OF THE CORRECT ANSWER IN THE SPACE AT THE RIGHT.*

Questions 1-7.

DIRECTIONS: Questions 1 through 7 refer to the passage that follows. Base your choice on the information in the passage *and on your own knowledge of science.*

In the days of sailing ships, when voyages were long and uncertain, provisions for many months were stored without refrigeration in the holds of the ships. Naturally no fresh or perishable foods could be included. Toward the end of particularly long voyages the crews of such ships became ill and often many died from scurvy. Many men, both scientific and otherwise, tried to devise a cure for scurvy. Among the latter was John Hall, a son-in-law of William Shakespeare, who cured some cases of scurvy by administering a sour brew made from scurvy grass and watercress.

The next step was the suggestion of William Harvey that scurvy could be prevented by giving the men lemon juice. He thought that the beneficial substance was the acid contained in the fruit.

The third step was taken by Dr. James Lind, an English naval surgeon, who performed the following experiment with 12 sailors all of whom were sick with scurvy: Each was given the same diet, except that four of the men received small amounts of dilute sulfuric acid, four others were given vinegar and the remaining four were given lemons. Only those who received the fruit recovered.

1. Credit for solving the problem described above belongs to

   A. HALL, because he first devised a cure for scurvy
   B. HARVEY, because he first proposed a solution of the problem
   C. LIND, because he proved the solution by means of an experiment
   D. both HARVEY and LIND, because they found that lemons are more effective than scurvy grass or watercress
   E. all three men, because each made some contribution

2. A good substitute for lemons in the treatment of scurvy is

   A. fresh eggs   B. tomato juice   C. cod-liver oil
   D. liver   E. whole-wheat bread

3. The number of control groups that Dr. Lind used in his experiment was

   A. one   B. two   C. three   D. four   E. none

4. A substance that will turn blue litmus red is

   A. aniline   B. lye   C. ice   D. vinegar   E. table salt

5. The hypothesis tested by Lind was:

   A. Lemons contain some substance not present in vinegar.
   B. Citric acid is the most effective treatment for scurvy.
   C. Lemons contain some unknown acid that will cure scurvy.
   D. Some specific substance, rather than acids in general, is needed to cure scurvy.
   E. The substance needed to cure scurvy is found only in lemons.

6. A problem that Lind's experiment did NOT solve was:

   A. Will citric acid alone cure scurvy?
   B. Will lemons cure scurvy?
   C. Will either sulfuric acid or vinegar cure scurvy?
   D. Are all substances that contain acids equally effective as a treatment for scurvy?
   E. Are lemons more effective than either vinegar or sulfuric acid in the treatment of scurvy?

7. The PRIMARY purpose of a controlled scientific experiment is to

   A. get rid of superstitions
   B. prove a hypothesis is correct
   C. disprove a theory that is false
   D. determine whether a hypothesis is true or false
   E. discover new facts

Questions 8-15.

DIRECTIONS: Questions 8 through 15 refer to the passage that follows. Base your choice on the information in the passage and *on your own knowledge of science*.

Photosynthesis is a complex process with many intermediate steps. Ideas differ greatly as to the details of these steps, but the general nature of the process and its outcome are well established. Water, usually from the soil, is conducted through the xylem of root, stem and leaf to the chlorophyl-containing cells of a leaf. In consequence of the abundance of water within the latter cells, their walls are saturated with water. Carbon dioxide, diffusing from the air through the stomata and into the intercellular spaces of the leaf, comes into contact with the water in the walls of the cells, which adjoin the intercellular spaces. The carbon dioxide becomes dissolved in the water in these walls, and in solution diffuses through the walls and the plasma membranes into the cells. By the agency of chlorphyl in the chloroplasts of the cells, the energy of light is transformed into chemical energy. This chemical energy is used to decompose the carbon dioxide and water, and the products of their decomposition are recombined into a new compound. The compound first formed is successively built up into more and more complex substances until finally a sugar is produced.

8. The union of carbon dioxide and water to form starch results in an excess of

   A. hydrogen   B. carbon   C. oxygen
   D. carbon monoxide   E. hydrogen peroxide

9. Synthesis of carbohydrates takes place

   A. in the stomata
   B. in the intercellular spaces of leaves
   C. in the walls of plant cells
   D. within the plasma membranes of plant cells
   E. within plant cells that contain chloroplasts

10. In the process of photosynthesis, chlorophyl acts as a   10.____

    A. carbohydrate   B. source of carbon dioxide
    C. catalyst   D. source of chemical energy
    E. plasma membrane

11. In which of the following places are there the GREATEST number of hours in which pho- 11.____
    tosynthesis can take place during the month of December?

    A. Buenos Aires, Argentina   B. Caracas, Venezuela
    C. Fairbanks, Alaska   D. Quito, Ecuador
    E. Calcutta, India

12. During photosynthesis, molecules of carbon dioxide enter the stomata of leaves because 12.____

    A. the molecules are already in motion
    B. they are forced through the stomata by the sun's rays
    C. chlorophyl attracts them
    D. a chemical change takes place in the stomata
    E. oxygen passes out through the stomata

13. Besides food manufacture, another useful result of photosynthesis is that it 13.____

    A. aids in removing poisonous gases from the air
    B. helps to maintain the existing proportion of gases in the air
    C. changes complex compounds into simpler compounds
    D. changes certain waste products into hydrocarbons
    E. changes chlorophyl into useful substances

14. A process that is ALMOST the exact reverse of photosynthesis is the 14.____

    A. rusting of iron   B. burning of wood
    C. digestion of starch   D. ripening of fruit
    E. storage of food in seeds

15. The leaf of the tomato plant will be unable to carry on photosynthesis if the 15.____

    A. upper surface of the leaf is coated with vaseline
    B. upper surface of the leaf is coated with lampblack
    C. lower surface of the leaf is coated with lard
    D. leaf is placed in an atmosphere of pure carbon dioxide
    E. entire leaf is coated with lime

Questions 16-24.

DIRECTIONS: Questions 16 through 24 refer to the passage that follows. Base your choice on the information in the passage and *on your own knowledge of science.*

The British pressure suit was made in two pieces and joined around the middle in contrast to the other suits, which were one-piece suits with a removable helmet. Oxygen was supplied through a tube, and a container of soda lime absorbed carbon dioxide and water vapor. The pressure was adjusted to a maximum of 2 1/2 pounds per square inch (130 millimeters) higher than the surrounding air. Since pure oxygen was used, this produced a partial pressure of 130 millimeters, which is sufficient to sustain the flier at any altitude.

Using this pressure suit, the British established a world's altitude record of 49,944 feet in 1936 and succeeded in raising it to 53,937 feet the following year. The pressure suit is a compromise solution to the altitude problem. Full sea-level pressure cannot be maintained, as the suit would be so rigid that the flier could not move arms or legs. Hence a pressure one-third to one-fifth that of sea level has been used. Because of these lower pressures, oxygen has been used to raise the partial pressure of alveolar oxygen to normal.

16. The MAIN constituent of air NOT admitted to the pressure suit described was

   A. oxygen   B. nitrogen   C. water vapor
   D. carbon dioxide   E. hydrogen

17. The pressure within the suit exceeded that of the surrounding air by an amount equal to 130 millimeters of

   A. mercury   B. water   C. air
   D. oxygen   E. carbon dioxide

18. The normal atmospheric pressure at sea level is

   A. 130 mm   B. 250 mm   C. 760 mm   D. 1000 mm   E. 1300 mm

19. The water vapor that was absorbed by the soda lime came from

   A. condensation
   B. the union of oxygen with carbon dioxide
   C. body metabolism
   D. the air within the pressure suit
   E. water particles in the upper air

20. The HIGHEST altitude that has been reached with the British pressure suit is about

   A. 130 miles   B. 2 1/2 miles   C. 6 miles   D. 10 miles
   E. 5 miles

21. If the pressure suit should develop a leak, the

   A. oxygen supply would be cut off
   B. suit would fill up with air instead of oxygen
   C. pressure within the suit would drop to zero
   D. pressure within the suit would drop to that of the surrounding air
   E. suit would become so rigid that the flier would be unable to move arms or legs

22. The reason why oxygen helmets are unsatisfactory for use in efforts to set higher altitude records is that

   A. it is impossible to maintain a tight enough fit at the neck
   B. oxygen helmets are too heavy
   C. they do not conserve the heat of the body as pressure suits do

D. if a parachute jump becomes necessary, it cannot be made while such a helmet is being worn
E. oxygen helmets are too rigid

23. The pressure suit is termed a compromise solution because

   A. it is not adequate for stratosphere flying
   B. aviators cannot stand sea-level pressure at high altitudes
   C. some suits are made in two pieces, others in one
   D. other factors than maintenance of pressure have to be accommodated
   E. full atmospheric pressure cannot be maintained at high altitudes

24. The passage implies that

   A. the air pressure at 49,944 feet is approximately the same as it is at 53,937 feet
   B. pressure cabin planes are not practical at extremely high altitudes
   C. a flier's oxygen requirement is approximately the same at high altitudes as it is at sea level
   D. one-piece pressure suits with removable helmets are unsafe
   E. a normal alveolar oxygen supply is maintained if the air pressure is between one-third and one-fifth that of sea level

25. If two 100-lb forces act concurrently so that their resultant is 50 lbs., the angle between them is which one of the following?

   A. Acute   B. Right   C. Obtuse   D. Straight   E. Oblique

26. The frequency of vibration of a string varies

   A. directly as the length
   B. directly as the square root of the tension
   C. inversely as the weight per unit length
   D. directly as the square root of the length
   E. directly as the length and inversely as the square foot of the tension

27. A 40 lb. force acting at an angle of 30° with a lever produces the same moment as a second force applied perpendicularly at the same point. The magnitude of this second force (in pounds) is

   A. 20   B. 35   C. 60   D. 80   E. 100

28. Assume that a simple pendulum has a period of one second. If the mass of the bob is doubled, and the length of the string is quadrupled, the new period (in seconds) is

   A. one   B. two   C. four   D. eight   E. sixteen

29. A given mass of an ideal gas is heated isothermally until it has a volume of 200 cm. If initially the gas had a volume of 100 cm^3 at a gauge pressure of 15 lb/in^2, the final gauge pressure (in pounds per square inch) will be CLOSEST to which one of the following?

   A. zero   B. 7.5   C. 15   D. 30   E. 60

30. A pulley with a mechanical advantage of two is used to lift a 500 lb. weight 20 ft. The potential energy of the weight (in ft.lb) increased

   A. 500   B. 5,000   C. 10,000   D. 20,000   E. 40,000

31. Of the following, the natural process which might require an energy input of about 10^{24} ergs/hour is

   A. the glow of a firefly
   B. a hurricane
   C. a bird's flight
   D. insolation per square foot at the equator
   E. an earthquake

32. If the molecules in a cylinder of oxygen and those in a cylinder of hydrogen have the same average speed, then

   A. both gases have the same temperature
   B. both gases have the same pressure
   C. the hydrogen has the higher temperature
   D. the oxygen has the higher temperature
   E. the hydrogen has the higher temperature when the oxygen has the lower temperature

33. Of the following, which condition exists in a perfectly inelastic collision?

   A. Neither momentum nor kinetic energy are conserved
   B. Both momentum and kinetic energy are conserved
   C. Momentum is conserved, but not kinetic energy
   D. Kinetic energy is conserved, but not momentum
   E. There is no relationship between momentum and kinetic energy

34. A simple series circuit consists of a cell, an ammeter, and a rheostat of resistance R. The ammeter reads 5 amps. When the resistance of the rheostat is increased by 2 ohms, the ammeter reading drops to 4 amps. The original resistance (in ohms) of the rheostat R is

   A. 2.5   B. 4.0   C. 8.0   D. 10.0   E. 12.0

35. A simple steam engine receives steam from the boiler at 180° C and exhausts directly into the air at 100° C. The upper limit of its thermal efficiency (in percent) is CLOSEST to which one of the following?

   A. 17.6   B. 28.0   C. 35.5   D. 80.0   E. 92.6

36. Two lamps need 50V and 2 amp each in order to operate at a desired brilliancy. If they are to be connected in series across a 120V line, the resistance (in ohms) of the rheostat that must be placed in series with the lamps needs to be

   A. 4   B. 10   C. 20   D. 100   E. 200

37. As the photon is a quantum in electromagnetic field theory, which one of the following is considered to be the quantum in the nuclear field?

   A. Neutrino   B. Electron   C. Meson   D. Neutron
   E. None of them

38. A 5 diopter lens has a focal length (in cm) CLOSEST to which one of the following? 38._____

    A. 1/5   B. 5   C. 20   D. 50   E. 100

39. The infra-red spectrometer has a prism that is GENERALLY made of which one of the following? 39._____

    A. Quartz   B. Glass   C. Sodium chloride
    D. Carbon disulfide E. Sodium disulfide

40. When an electron moves with a speed equal to 4/5 that of light, the ratio of its mass to its rest mass is which one of the following? 40._____

    A. 5/4   B. 5/3   C. 25/9   D. 25/16   E. 4/5

41. A pulley on an electric motor turns clockwise. A crossed belt turns a much larger pulley on a feed grinder. The pulley on the feed grinder turns 41._____

    A. clockwise and slower than the one on the motor
    B. counterclockwise and slower than the one on the motor
    C. clockwise and faster than the one on the motor
    D. counterclockwise and faster than the one on the motor
    E. clockwise and at the same speed as the one on the motor

42. The sprocket wheels and chain of a bicycle increase the 42._____

    A. power of the rider
    B. force applied to the rear wheel
    C. force applied to the road
    D. speed of the rear wheel
    E. energy output of the rider

43. Soda pop rises along a soda straw into one's mouth because 43._____

    A. nature abhors a vacuum
    B. there is capillary action in the straw
    C. the air pressure on the pop is greater than the pressure in one's mouth
    D. the vacuum in one's mouth pulls up the pop
    E. the carbon dioxide pressure in the pop forces it upwards

44. Which of the following principles BEST explains the propulsion of a jet plane? 44._____

    A. Every action has an equal and opposite reaction
    B. Energy can be neither created nor destroyed
    C. Every effect has a cause
    D. If pressure is applied to a confined gas, the volume of the gas will decrease
    E. Compression of a gas produces heat

45. To make an airplane bank on a left turn, the left 45._____

    A. elevator is raised and the right elevator is lowered
    B. pedal is pushed and the right pedal is pulled
    C. aileron is raised and the right aileron is lowered
    D. stabilizer is raised and the right stabilizer is lowered
    E. wing is tilted upward and the right wing is tilted downward

46. A ship entering a fresh-water river from the ocean will sink deeper because   46._____

    A. salt water has greater viscosity than fresh water
    B. salt holds objects up
    C. a cubic foot of salt water weighs more than a cubic foot of fresh water
    D. surface tension is greater in the river
    E. oceans are deeper

47. The fuel in the cylinder of a Diesel engine is ignited by   47._____

    A. an electric spark   B. a pilot light   C. the injector
    D. a supercharger   E. the heat of compression

48. A three-element vacuum tube in an electric circuit   48._____

    A. generates signals of increased voltage
    B. amplifies the grid bias
    C. controls the electron flow in the circuit
    D. rectifies the B-battery output
    E. increases the signal frequency

49. Some highways are lighted at night by lamps that produce a golden-yellow light. This color is due to the passage of electricity through the vapor of   49._____

    A. argon   B. helium   C. mercury   D. nitrogen   E. sodium

50. A fluorescent lamp produces light by the   50._____

    A. ionization of the Heaviside layer
    B. glowing of an incandescent filament
    C. production of X-rays
    D. action of infrared rays, which heat the glass
    E. action of ultraviolet rays on a mineral coating on the glass

---

KEY (CORRECT ANSWERS)

1. E	11. A	21. D	31. B	41. B
2. B	12. A	22. D	32. D	42. D
3. B	13. B	23. E	33. C	43. C
4. D	14. B	24. C	34. C	44. A
5. D	15. C	25. C	35. A	45. C
6. A	16. B	26. B	36. B	46. C
7. D	17. A	27. A	37. C	47. E
8. C	18. C	28. B	38. C	48. C
9. E	19. C	29. A	39. C	49. E
10. C	20. D	30. C	40. B	50. E

EXAMINATION SECTION
TEST 1

DIRECTIONS: Each question or incomplete statement is followed by several suggested answers or completions. Select the one that BEST answers the question or completes the statement. *PRINT THE LETTER OF THE CORRECT ANSWER IN THE SPACE AT THE RIGHT.*

Questions 1-9.

DIRECTIONS: Questions 1 through 9 are based on the following passage.

Astronomers have long argued whether a tenth planet, Planet X, exists in the solar system. Two astronomers presented their opinions. Astronomer 1 argued that Planet X does not exist, and Astronomer 2 argued that Planet X does exist.

Astronomer 1

The 4 terrestrial (smaller) planets - Mercury, Venus, Mars, and Earth - orbit near the Sun and consist mainly of heavier, denser elements. The 4 giant planets - Jupiter, Saturn, Uranus, and Neptune -orbit farther from the Sun and contain mostly lighter elements, which are gaseous on Earth. The ninth planet, Pluto, is smaller than the Earth, and its orbit is inclined from the common orbital plane of the other planets. Therefore, Pluto probably did not originate within the solar system, but was captured from outside. It is very unlikely that the solar system would capture 2 planets. It is also unlikely that Pluto could have been captured between the orbits of Neptune and Planet X if Planet X had been formed with the rest of the solar system.

Some astronomers cite the orbital deviation of comets to support the theory that Planet X exists. But the force of solar radiation or collisions with meteoroids could account for these deviations. Deviation in Neptune's orbit has also been used to try to demonstrate Planet X's existence. But undiscovered causes may account for this deviation. Finally, Planet X should also have caused deviation in Pluto's orbit. However, none has been discovered.

Astronomer 2

Even if Pluto had been captured, that would still not disprove the existence of Planet X. Pluto may once have been a moon of Planet X or Neptune. Planet X probably is 3 times more massive than Saturn and 1 1/2 times farther from the Sun than is Pluto. Only such a massive object could cause comets and the planet Neptune to deviate from their orbits. Finally, Pluto has completed only 1/4 of its orbit since its discovery. Astronomers may yet find a deviation in Pluto's orbit that would support the theory that Planet X exists.

1. According to Astronomer 2, if Planet X existed, it would PROBABLY be less massive than

   A. Venus
   B. Earth
   C. Mars
   D. none of the above planets

2. A comet would experience the GREATEST force of radiation when it was closest to

   A. the Sun
   B. the giant planets
   C. Pluto
   D. Planet X

3. Astronomer 1 implies that the 4 terrestrial and the 4 giant planets were formed

   A. at the center of the Sun
   B. in the immediate neighborhood of the Sun
   C. outside the solar system
   D. in the order of their distances from the Sun, from farthest to nearest

4. Concerning the orbital deviation of comets, Astronomers 1 and 2 DISAGREE about the

   A. existence of the deviations
   B. magnitude of the deviations
   C. nature of the force causing the deviations
   D. existence of the force of radiation

5. If a deviation were observed in the orbit of Pluto, the astronomer that would be MOST seriously challenged would be Astronomer _____ because such deviation would _____ .

   A. 1; have to be caused by meteor showers
   B. 1; have to be caused by a massive object
   C. 2; have to be caused by Neptune
   D. 2; prove Pluto is a captured planet

6. Jupiter and Mercury have similar

   A. orbital radii
   B. chemical compositions
   C. masses
   D. planes of orbit

7. On the basis of Astronomer 2's arguments, one could infer that a failure to view Planet X with a telescope could be due to the fact that Planet X is

   A. obscured by swarms of comets located far from the Sun
   B. hidden in Pluto's shadow
   C. located in a part of the sky that has not yet been carefully examined
   D. gaseous and absorbs light

8. Astronomer 2 implies that the deviation in the path of a comet would be caused by

   A. magnetic force
   B. gravitational force
   C. radiation from the Sun
   D. collision with another body

9. In the solar system, gravitational force is caused by the
   I. Sun
   II. giant planets
   III. terrestrial planets
   The CORRECT answer is:

   A. I only
   B. II only
   C. I and II
   D. All of the above

Questions 10-18.

DIRECTIONS: Questions 10 through 18 are based on the following passage.

To design an aircraft that can fly, engineers must solve certain basic problems. Today, engineers have computers and a large pool of knowledge to aid in the design of sophisticated aircraft. But the Wright brothers, Orville and Wilbur, used only a basic knowledge of physics and simple experiments to build the first powered aircraft, the Wright Flyer.

The Wrights hypothesized that an airplane must have a wing to generate *lift,* the upward force that offsets the weight of the airplane. The lift of a wing depends upon the area of the wing, the airspeed of the wing, the density of the air, and the *angle of attack* (the angle the wing makes with its direction of flight). But a moving wing also generates *drag,* the frictional force that resists movement. Drag increases as lift and airspeed increase. To overcome drag and to provide velocity to create lift, an airplane must generate *thrust,* the forward force provided in some aircraft by a propeller connected to an engine. To fly at a steady speed at a constant height, an airplane must maintain a balance among lift, weight, drag, and thrust. The Wrights used 2 wings in a biplane arrangement to provide lift and developed a light but powerful aluminum engine to create thrust.

Changing the direction of flight poses further problems. Simply moving the nose of an airplane to one side or the other will cause the airplane to make a broad skid turn. Its wings must *bank,* or tilt, in the direction of the turn before the airplane will change direction quickly. An airplane can be made to tip its nose up or down without climbing or diving by moving the *elevator,* a much smaller wing. This is done by changing the airspeed and thrust while increasing the angle of attack.

The Wrights made the Flyer bank by using cables that actually bent the wings. The Wrights believed that an aircraft must be unstable to change direction. They reasoned that the force necessary to turn a stable aircraft would be much greater than the force required to turn an unstable one. To make the Flyer unstable, the Wrights placed the elevators in front of the wings. The pilot had to correct any change in direction constantly or the change would rapidly increase. Later inventors learned that stable aircraft can easily change direction. As a result, modern airplanes are much simpler to control.

10. The forces acting on the airplane in flight are shown below.

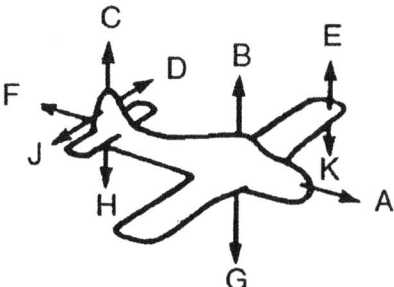

Which of these forces would have to be equal to each other in order to prevent the banking of the wings?

A. A and F
B. B and G
C. C and H
D. E and K

11. If the Wrights had wanted the Flyer to be stable, they PROBABLY would have

    A. placed the elevators behind the wings
    B. used 1 wing instead of 2
    C. added weight to the airplane
    D. increased the power of the engine

12. A conventional airplane that can fly at very low airspeeds MUST have a large

    A. wing area
    B. propeller
    C. amount of weight
    D. amount of drag

13. Both airplane and steamships use propellers. This fact indicates that both seawater and air

    A. have similar densities
    B. have similar chemical properties
    C. expand when heated
    D. flow readily under pressure

14. A certain modern aircraft with an engine approximately as powerful as that of the Wright Flyer can reach much greater speeds than the Flyer could.
    This difference in speed is due PRIMARILY to the fact that the modern aircraft has

    A. less drag
    B. greater drag
    C. greater lift
    D. greater weight

15. Which description of the forces acting upon a rocket rising vertically through the air must be TRUE?

    A. Drag is directed horizontally.
    B. Thrust is directed vertically.
    C. Thrust equals drag.
    D. Drag equals weight.

16. All winged aircraft have altitudes beyond which they cannot climb.
    This altitude limitation is due to the fact that as altitude increases, there is a decrease in

    A. drag
    B. gravity
    C. air density
    D. air temperature

17. An aircraft whose wings are much shorter than the length of the airplane was PROBABLY designed to

    A. carry large loads
    B. be unstable
    C. fly at high speeds
    D. fly at high altitudes

18. The fact that many aircraft can fly both upside down and rightside up demonstrates that lift depends upon

    A. drag
    B. the angle of attack
    C. banking the wings
    D. the weight of the airplane

Questions 19-33.

DIRECTIONS: Questions 19 through 33 are NOT based on a reading passage. You are to answer these questions on the basis of your knowledge in the natural sciences.

19.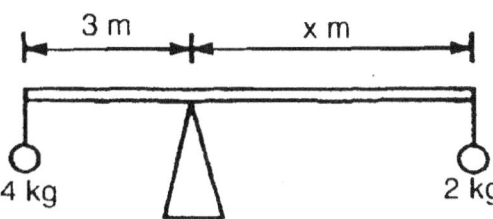

A uniform board of negligible mass is supported as shown above. A mass of 4 kilograms (kg) is suspended at one end, 3 meters from the point of support. A mass of 2 kilograms is suspended at the other end, x meters from the point of support.
If the board does NOT tilt, what is the length, in meters (m), of x?

A. 4   B. 6   C. 8   D. 12

20. A marble chip ($CaCO_3$) is dissolved in excess hydrochloric acid (HCl), and a gas is produced.
When the solution is evaporated, a white solid remains.
What is this solid?

A. Carbon (C)
B. Carbonic acid (H_2CO_3)
C. Calcium chloride ($CaCl_2$)
D. Calcium hydride (CaH_2)

21. A student places a cloth wick over the bulb of a thermometer, moistens the wick with water, and whirls the thermometer in the air.
The student is gathering data to calculate the
I. air pressure
II. wind speed
III. relative humidity
The CORRECT answer is:

A. I only   B. III only
C. I and II   D. II and III

22. Which of these structures prevent MOST plant cells from bursting in a hypotonic solution?

A. Chloroplasts   B. Cell walls
C. Lysosomes   D. Ribosomes

23. The more complex plants (ferns, gymnosperms, flowering plants) can achieve a larger size and a more complicated organ structure than the less complex plants (algae, mosses, liverworts) because the more complex plants

A. have vascular systems   B. contain chloroplasts
C. are capable of mitosis   D. have cell walls

24. Two objects of the same volume are placed in 2 separate containers containing clear, colorless liquids. One object sinks to the bottom, but the other floats. Which conclusion concerning the densities of the objects and liquids could validly be made WITHOUT conducting further experiments?

    A. One of the objects has a greater density than the other.
    B. One of the liquids has a greater density than the other.
    C. The object that sinks has a greater density than the liquid it is in.
    D. The 2 objects and the 2 liquids are all of different densities.

25. Which of these facts does NOT support the theory of continental drift?

    A. The distance between North America and Europe increases yearly by a small amount.
    B. Igneous rocks of the seafloor increase in age from both sides of the mid-Atlantic ridge.
    C. Newly formed volcanic islands quickly become populated with living organisms.
    D. Coal has been found in Antarctica.

26. Which of these characteristics is NOT a typical mammalian feature?

    A. Body hair
    B. Three bones in the middle ear
    C. Internal fertilization
    D. Two-chambered heart

27. Suppose a membrane bag filled with iodine solution is placed in a beaker containing a starch solution. A blue-black color forms in the solution in the beaker, but NOT in the solution in the bag.
    One can validly conclude that the membrane bag was

    A. impermeable to both starch and iodine
    B. impermeable to starch but permeable to iodine
    C. permeable to starch but impermeable to iodine
    D. permeable to both starch and iodine

28. A student measures the tension on a certain string and the frequency at which it vibrates. The resulting data are displayed in the table below:

Tension (newtons)	Frequency (cycles per second)
4	200
9	300
16	400

    Which equation accurately describes the relationship between string tension (T) and frequency (f)?
    f =

    A. $100\sqrt{T}$
    B. $\dfrac{100}{T}$
    C. $100T$
    D. $100T^2$

29. The noble gas neon is essentially chemically inert because its atoms   29.____

    A. form diatomic molecules
    B. bond together with triple covalent bonds
    C. bond together with highly charged ionic bonds
    D. have completely filled electron shells

30. Carbohydrates must be broken down into sugars before they can be absorbed by the human body.   30.____
    Which of these compounds does the body use to catalzye these reactions?

    A. Amino acids   B. Fats
    C. Hormones   D. Enzymes

31. Electrically neutral atoms of the Group IA elements, such as lithium, sodium, and potassium, all have equal numbers of   31.____

    A. protons   B. neutrons
    C. filled electron shells   D. valence electrons

32. An element with which of these electron configurations would be MOST reactive?   32.____

    A. $1s^1$ B. $1s^2 2s\, 2p$
    C. $1s^2 2s^2 2p^6$ D. $1s^2 2s^2 2p^6 3s^2 3p^6$

33. If a 2.0 liter sample of liquid water at 100 Celsius is mixed with 1.0 liter of liquid water at 0.0 Celsius, what would be the APPROXIMATE temperature of the mixture, in degrees Celsius?   33.____

    A. 33   B. 50   C. 67   D. 75

Questions 34-43.

DIRECTIONS: Questions 34 through 43 are based on the following passage.

All organisms exchange gases with their environments. Gases can enter or leave organisms only by passive diffusion across respiratory membranes. Whatever the life form, gases must be dissolved in the liquid covering the respiratory membrane before they can enter the organism.

Gas exchange surfaces in higher animals are generally formed by *evagination* - outward folding - or *invagination* - inward folding - of body surfaces. Aquatic animals usually have evaginated surfaces, such as gills. Oxygenated water constantly bathes these evaginated surfaces. As a bony fish swims, it forces water over its gills by opening and closing its mouth and gill flaps. Other aquatic forms have other methods of moving water over their gas exchange surfaces.

Land animals typically have invaginated gas exchange surfaces. The *tracheal system* of an insect is composed of a series of invaginated tubes leading from *spiracles* - openings on the insect's body - directly to the insect's cells. No cell is more than 1 or 2 cell layers away from the ending of a tracheal tube. Thus, oxygen diffuses directly into the cells instead of being transported by blood. The mammalian lung is another type of invaginated gas exchange surface. The lung is a highly branched series of invaginated tubes ending in sacs called *alveoli*. Each alveolus is surrounded by a network of capillaries. Oxygen in the alveoli dissolves in the moisture on the alveolar membranes and diffuses into blood cells in the capillaries.

There are exceptions to the general rule that aquatic organisms have evaginated gas exchange surfaces and land organisms have invaginated gas exchange surfaces. Sea cucumbers, for instance, have invaginated tubes that branch off the anal pouch. Water pumped into and out of the anal opening brings dissolved oxygen to the sea cucumber's respiratory membranes.

34. Individuals of certain fish species will die if prevented from moving through the water. The MOST likely reason why members of these species must keep moving is to

   A. keep their gills from invaginating
   B. supply energy for active transport of gases across respiratory membranes
   C. maintain pressure inside their tracheal tubes
   D. maintain a flow of water over their gills

35. Frogs can exchange gases through both their lungs and their

   A. hearts　　　　　　　　　　　B. intestines
   C. trqcheal tubes　　　　　　　D. skins

36. The hollow body of the hydra, a small aquatic organism, is a cylinder 2 cells thick. The hydra PROBABLY exchanges gases through

   A. gills
   B. sea cucumber-like tubes
   C. its entire body surface
   D. lungs

37. Crayfish have a pair of flat appendages located just in front of the gills. These appendages move back and forth continuously.
   To effectively exchange gases, crayfish, therefore, do NOT have to

   A. depend upon the passive diffusion of gases
   B. pump blood through their gills
   C. maintain a constant flow of water through their gills
   D. constantly move through the water

38. Which aquatic animal exchanges gases through an invaginated surface?

   A. Shark　　　B. Whale　　　C. Clam　　　D. Lobster

39. A certain vertebrate changes from an aquatic adolescent into a terrestrial adult. During this metamorphosis, the animal's gas exchange system would MOST likely

   A. change from gills to lungs
   B. change from tracheal tubes to lungs
   C. remain unchanged as tracheal tubes
   D. remain unchanged as gills

40. Larval tiger salamanders growing in iodine-deficient water never reach the adult stage. Which of these gas exchange surfaces would be used by these larval salamanders for respiration?
   I. Gills
   II. Lungs
   III. Tracheal tubes

   The CORRECT answer is:

   A. I only
   B. II only
   C. III only
   D. I and III

41. A common feature of all gas exchange surfaces is

   A. a branched structure
   B. moisture
   C. the presence of capillaries
   D. the presence of tracheal tubes

42. A decrease in the rate at which a certain gas enters an organism could be caused by a(n)

   A. *increase* in the organism's metabolic rate
   B. *increase* in the amount of energy available for active transport
   C. *decrease* in the partial pressure of the gas in the environment
   D. *increase* in the partial pressure of the gas in the environment

43. Compared to concentrations of oxygen and carbon dioxide in the air, blood entering the lungs must have a(n) _____ concentration of _____.

   A. higher; oxygen
   B. equal; oxygen
   C. higher; carbon dioxide
   D. equal; carbon dioxide

Questions 44-50.

DIRECTIONS: Questions 44 through 50 are based on the following passage.

Color can be a useful tool in laboratory experiments. The absorption or emission of certain ranges of light wavelengths by ions or molecules causes color. The principal colors of light are red, orange, yellow, green, blue, and violet, each of which is associated with certain wavelengths. Other colors can be formed by the absorption or emission of combinations of these wavelengths.

Absorption of characteristic wavelengths of light by particles of *solutes* (dissolved substances) gives solutions their colors. Solution color is often affected by chemical reactions among solutes. *Oxidation-reduction reactions,* in which electrons are transferred among solute particles, can cause color changes. The addition of an acid or base to a solution also may produce a different color. An aqueous cobalt(II) chloride solution, for example, is red. In general, if an acid is added, the solution remains red. However, the addition of a base turns the solution blue and cloudy as cobalt(II) hydroxide forms and precipitates.

The colors of certain organic compounds known as *indicators* can be used to mark changes in the acidity of a solution. Some of the indicator molecules ionize in solution, and the resulting ions absorb different wavelengths of light than do the molecules. Since the ratio of ions to molecules depends upon the acidity of the solution, the color of the solution changes when the acidity reaches a certain known value.

In one method of *acid-base titration,* indicators are used to measure the concentration of a solution. A drop of indicator is added to a solution whose *molarity* (molar concentration, in moles per liter) is known. Small amounts of the solution of unknown concentration are measured into the known solution until the indicator changes color, marking neutralization. Using the molarity and volume of the known solution, the volume of the unknown solution used in the reaction, and the reaction equation, a chemist can determine the molarity of the unknown solution.

For example, suppose 500 milliliters of a sodium hydroxide solution of unknown concentration just causes the indicator in 1 liter of 0.01 M (moles per liter) sulfuric acid (H_2SO_4) to change color. Sodium hydroxide (NaOH) and sulfuric acid react according to the equation

$$H_2SO_4 + 2NaOH \rightarrow Na_2SO_4 + 2H_2O$$

The equation shows that twice as many moles of sodium hydroxide as sulfuric acid were used in the reaction. Since the sulfuric acid contained 0.01 mole of H_2O_4, all of which was neutralized, 0.02 mole of sodium hydroxide must have been used. The concentration of the sodium hydroxide solution is, therefore,

$$\frac{0.02 \text{ mole}}{500 \text{ milliliters}} \times \frac{1,000 \text{ milliliters}}{1 \text{ liter}} = 0.04M$$

44. Nitric acid (HNO_3 in aqueous solution) is colorless. An aqueous solution of nickel(II) nitrate [$Ni(NO_3)_2$], is green.
These facts support the conclusion that the green color of nickel(II) nitrate is caused by _____ ions.

 A. nitrate   B. nickel(II)
 C. nitrogen   D. oxygen

44.____

45. Which of these procedures would distinguish blue light caused by emission from blue light caused by absorption?

 A. Projecting the light through a colored solution
 B. Reflecting the light from a mirror
 C. Reflecting the light from the surface of water
 D. None of the above

45.____

46. If a drop of phenolphthalein is added to a beaker of aqueous sodium hydroxide, the solution becomes deep red. The addition of hydrogen chloride eventually causes the solution to become colorless.
This information supports the conclusion about phenolphthalein that it

 A. forms a precipitate when added to a base
 B. emits red light when added to a base
 C. is useful as an indicator in acid-base titration
 D. is decomposed by strong acids

46.____

47. Hydrochloric acid (HCl) and potassium hydroxide (KOH) react according to the equation shown below:

   HCl + KOH → KCl + H$_2$O

   Suppose 500 milliliters of 0.20 M KOH solution is exactly neutralized by 250 milliliters of HCl solution. What is the molarity of the HC1 solution?

   A. 0.10 B. 0.20 C. 0.40 D. 0.80

48. As water is added to a red cobalt(II) chloride solution, the solution color changes to pink. Which of these explanations of this color change is CORRECT?

   A. Less light is absorbed per unit volume of solution.
   B. Cobalt(II) and chloride ions bond with water molecules and absorb different wavelengths.
   C. Chloride ions absorb heat from water and emit pink light.
   D. Excess water causes cobalt(II) and chloride ions to bond, emitting pink light.

49. A certain indicator is colorless in acid and neutral solutions but turns blue in basic solutions. Suppose it is added to a solution, which remains colorless.
   The addition of which substance will change the color of the indicator?

   A. Ammonia
   B. Carbon dioxide
   C. Hydrogen fluoride
   D. Sulfur dioxide

50. The red color of a cobalt(II) chloride solution is caused by the cobalt(II) ion's

   A. emission of red wavelengths
   B. emission of all wavelengths except red
   C. absorption of red wavelengths
   D. absorption of all wavelengths except red

KEY (CORRECT ANSWERS)

1. D	11. A	21. B	31. D	41. B
2. A	12. A	22. B	32. A	42. C
3. B	13. D	23. A	33. C	43. C
4. C	14. A	24. C	34. D	44. B
5. B	15. B	25. C	35. D	45. D
6. D	16. C	26. D	36. C	46. C
7. C	17. C	27. B	37. D	47. C
8. B	18. B	28. A	38. B	48. A
9. D	19. B	29. D	39. A	49. A
10. D	20. C	30. D	40. A	50. D

EXAMINATION SECTION
TEST 1

DIRECTIONS: Each question or incomplete statement is followed by several suggested answers or completions. Select the one that BEST answers the question or completes the statement. *PRINT THE LETTER OF THE CORRECT ANSWER IN THE SPACE AT THE RIGHT.*

1. Respiration in plants occurs
    A. only on cloudy days
    B. only in the night
    C. only in the daytime
    D. all the time

2. The complex chemical ATP is necessary to produce
    A. fats
    B. sugars
    C. proteins
    D. amino acids

3. A medicine obtained from the bark of the cinchona tree is
    A. atabrine
    B. pentaquine
    C. chloroquine
    D. quinine

4. A radioactive element used to study photosynthesis in green plants is
    A. I^{131}
    B. C^{14}
    C. N^{16}
    D. U^{233}

5. The selectivity of a cell depends upon the
    A. cell membrane
    B. nucleus
    C. cytoplasm
    D. mitochondria

6. The zoologist who helped formulate the cell theory was
    A. Schleiden
    B. Hooke
    C. Purkinje
    D. Schwann

7. The brown spots on the back of fern fronds produce
    A. pollen
    B. spores
    C. scales
    D. seeds

8. Plants without true roots, stems, or leaves are called
    A. bryophytes
    B. spermatophytes
    C. thallophytes
    D. pteridophytes

9. Of the following, the CLOSEST biological relative of the whale is the
    A. shark
    B. toad
    C. crocodile
    D. horse

10. The process LEAST likely to result in vitamin loss is
    A. bleaching celery
    B. refining flour
    C. quick freezing fruits
    D. peeling vegetables

11. A trait determined by two identical alleles is said to be
    A. homologous
    B. analogous
    C. heterozygous
    D. homozygous

12. The nutrient that produces the LARGEST number of calories per gram of weight is

    A. protein B. starch C. carbohydrate D. fat

13. A method used to condition the soil by spreading straw, manure, or peat moss over it is

    A. fallowing B. terracing C. leaching D. mulching

14. The plant that acts as an alternate host for the wheat rust is

    A. gooseberry B. white pine
    C. red cedar D. barberry

15. In the process of respiration in a plant,

    A. potential energy is stored
    B. chlorophyll is necessary
    C. stored food is utilized
    D. protein is synthesized

16. The insect that feeds on the cottony cushion scale is the

    A. Ladybird bettle B. Boll weevil
    C. Tachina fly D. Hessian fly

17. Food made in the leaves moves to all parts of a green plant through the

    A. stomates B. phloem C. pith D. xylem

18. Deamination of proteins occurs MAINLY in the

    A. small intestine B. liver
    C. spleen D. pancreas

19. The chemical that plays a part in the passage of nerve impulses across the space between two connecting neurons is

    A. auxin B. colchicine
    C. reserpine D. acetylcholine

20. The gathering of white blood cells around bacteria is an example of

    A. thigmotropism B. chemotropism
    C. geotropism D. hydrotropism

21. The Islets of Langerhans are located in the

    A. testis B. pancreas C. pituitary D. thyroid

22. The adrenal cortex is stimulated to secrete cortisone by

    A. ATP B. ACTH C. 2, 4-D D. PAS

23. Liquid wastes are carried from the kidneys to the urinary bladder by the

    A. ureters B. urethras
    C. oviducts D. Fallopian tubes

24. The part of the brain that controls the breathing rate is the
    A. medulla
    B. cerebrum
    C. cerebellum
    D. hypothalamus

25. The chemicals that cause clumping of the erythrocytes in the blood are
    A. platelets
    B. red corpuscles
    C. white corpuscles
    D. plasma

26. An organism with an *open circuit* system of circulation is the
    A. frog
    B. earthworm
    C. crayfish
    D. fish

27. The heart chamber that pumps blood to the aorta is the
    A. right auricle
    B. right ventricle
    C. left auricle
    D. left ventricle

28. The substances that are absorbed into the lacteals of the villi are
    A. amino acids
    B. vitamins
    C. simple sugars
    D. fatty acids

29. A chemical that has been used with great success in the treatment of tuberculosis is
    A. isoniazid
    B. chloromycetin
    C. sulfanilamide
    D. radioactive phosphorus

30. Ringworm disease is caused by a
    A. lichen
    B. roundworm
    C. segmented worm
    D. fungus

31. The organism that causes typhus fever is a(n)
    A. fungus
    B. Rickettsia
    C. bacterium
    D. virus

32. Emotional behavior is controlled in the
    A. hypothalamus
    B. cerebrum
    C. cerebellum
    D. medulla

33. In a given sample of blood, clumping occurred with both A serum and B serum. The blood type was
    A. A
    B. B
    C. O
    D. AB

34. Of the following vitamins, the one that does NOT aid in cellular oxidation is
    A. thiamin
    B. niacin
    C. ascorbic acid
    D. riboflavin

35. The cyton of a motor neuron is found in the
    A. posterior root ganglion
    B. anterior root ganglion
    C. gray matter of the spinal cord
    D. white matter of the spinal cord

36. An instrument that records the electrical impulses developed in the brain is the

    A. kymograph
    B. electrocardiograph
    C. polygraph
    D. electroencephalograph

37. The relationship between clover plants and nitrogen-fixing bacteria is a form of

    A. parasitism
    B. saprophytism
    C. commensalism
    D. symbiosis

38. The number of pairs of cranial nerves in man is

    A. 12   B. 31   C. 48   D. 206

39. Water pollination occurs in the

    A. water lily
    B. corn
    C. spruce
    D. duckweed

40. A vegetative structure that consists of an underground stem surrounded by storage-leaves is a

    A. slip   B. rhizome   C. bulb   D. tuber

41. If a planarium is cut in half, each part will grow eventually into a complete organism. This process of forming a new organism is called

    A. conjugation
    B. parthenogenesis
    C. meiosis
    D. regeneration

42. Passive immunity GENERALLY lasts a

    A. few weeks
    B. few months
    C. few years
    D. lifetime

43. Septic tanks are used in waste disposal to

    A. break down solid wastes
    B. dilute sewage
    C. aerate sewage
    D. filter sewage

44. The development of the polio vaccine was made possible, in part, by the discovery that the polio viruses could be cultured in test tubes on one of the following organs of Old World monkeys:

    A. Liver
    B. Thyroid gland
    C. Kidney
    D. Lung

45. The scientist who discovered streptomycin was

    A. Enders   B. Fleming   C. Florey   D. Waksman

46. A sex-linked disease in man is

    A. leukemia
    B. anemia
    C. hemophilia
    D. erythroblastosis fetalis

47. Destruction of the red blood cells of a developing embryo may occur when the embryo is Rh _____ and the mother is Rh _____.

   A. positive; positive
   B. positive; negative
   C. negative; negative
   D. negative; positive

48. The scientist who FIRST used the word mutation to describe changes that he found in the evening primrose plant was

   A. Morgan   B. Muller   C. DeVries   D. Mendel

49. The study of the functioning of living organisms is called

   A. anatomy   B. pathology   C. ecology   D. physiology

50. The fact that a white guinea pig resulted from a cross between two hybrid black guinea pigs illustrates the law of

   A. segregation
   B. dominance
   C. linkage
   D. independent assortment

KEY (CORRECT ANSWERS)

1. D	11. D	21. B	31. B	41. D
2. B	12. D	22. B	32. A	42. A
3. D	13. D	23. A	33. D	43. A
4. B	14. D	24. A	34. C	44. C
5. A	15. C	25. D	35. C	45. D
6. D	16. A	26. C	36. D	46. C
7. B	17. B	27. D	37. D	47. B
8. C	18. B	28. D	38. A	48. C
9. D	19. D	29. A	39. D	49. D
10. C	20. B	30. D	40. C	50. A

TEST 2

DIRECTIONS: Each question or incomplete statement is followed by several suggested answers or completions. Select the one that BEST answers the question or completes the statement. *PRINT THE LETTER OF THE CORRECT ANSWER IN THE SPACE AT THE RIGHT.*

1. When a blue Andalusian rooster is crossed with a blue Andalusian hen, the phenotypic ratio expected among the offspring will be

    A. 100% blue
    B. 50% black and 50% white
    C. 75% black and 25% white
    D. 25% white, 25% black, 50% blue

    1.____

2. A vitamin that contains cobalt as part of its chemical structure is vitamin

    A. A   B. B_2 C. B_{12} D. C

    2.____

3. The two-layered cup stage that forms during cleavage is called the

    A. morula   B. gastrula   C. blastula   D. mesoderm

    3.____

4. The one term that includes all the others is

    A. equational division   B. gamete
    C. maturation   D. reduction division

    4.____

5. Organizers are chemicals that influence

    A. differentiation   B. mitosis
    C. fertilization   D. maturation

    5.____

6. The developing embryo of a mammal is protected by a liquid-filled sac called the

    A. placenta   B. amnion   C. uterus   D. allantois

    6.____

7. The seedless orange is propagated by

    A. self-pollination   B. cross-pollination
    C. hybridization   D. grafting

    7.____

8. One similarity between reflexes and habits is that they are BOTH

    A. inborn acts   B. autonomic acts
    C. learned acts   D. automatic

    8.____

9. The MOST ancient of the following prehistoric men is

    A. Heidelberg   B. Neanderthal
    C. Pithecantropus   D. Cro-Magnon

    9.____

10. The theory of *Use and Disuse* was developed by

    A. Weismann   B. Darwin   C. Wallace   D. Lamarck

    10.____

11. The micturating membrane in man is an example of a(n)
    A. mutation
    B. vestigial structure
    C. malformation
    D. embryonic structure

12. The LATEST of the geological eras is called the
    A. cenozoic
    B. paleozoic
    C. proterozoic
    D. mesozoic

13. Liquids are transported through stems and roots by the
    A. epidermis
    B. cortex
    C. vascular bundles
    D. pith

14. An animal that is PROBABLY a link between the fish and amphibia is the
    A. archeopteryx
    B. coelacanth
    C. trilobite
    D. lamprey

15. The hormone that stimulates the change of glycogen to glucose in the liver is
    A. insulin
    B. progestin
    C. cortin
    D. adrenin

16. The haploid chromosome number in the fruit fly, Drosophila, is
    A. 4
    B. 8
    C. 24
    D. 48

17. The plant in which seed dispersal by animals occurs is the
    A. cherry
    B. coconut
    C. witch hazel
    D. milkweed

18. Blood tissue differentiates from the primary germ layer known as the
    A. endoderm
    B. endosperm
    C. mesoderm
    D. ectoderm

19. Of the following types of tissue, the one which is NOT classified as connective tissue is
    A. blood
    B. bone
    C. cartilage
    D. tendon

20. A chrysalis is a
    A. pupa case
    B. nymph
    C. larva
    D. cocoon

21. The one term that includes all the others is _____ plant.
    A. herbaceous
    B. flowering
    C. spermatophyte
    D. annual

22. Nitrogen from the air is made available to plants by
    A. decay
    B. fixation
    C. denitrification
    D. nitrate bacteria

23. The series of muscular waves of contraction in the alimentary canal is called
    A. pylorus
    B. peristalsis
    C. symbiosis
    D. parthenogenesis

24. The corals belong to the phylum

    A. Mollusca B. Porifera
    C. Arthropoda D. Coelenterata

25. Three of the following substances are narcotics. The one that is NOT is

    A. chlorpromazine B. nicotine
    C. morphine D. cocaine

26. Hydrogen sulfide is USUALLY prepared in the laboratory by the action of

    A. hydrogen on hot sulfur
    B. hydrochloric acid on ferrous sulfide
    C. acid on sulfite
    D. sulfuric acid on copper

27. An unknown gas dissolves readily in water. The water solution turns red litmus blue. The gas reacts with hydrogen chloride gas, forming white fumes.
    The unknown gas is PROBABLY

    A. nitric oxide B. ammonia
    C. sulfur dioxide D. hydrogen sulfide

28. Of the following, the one whose water solution will be basic in reaction is 0.1 molar

    A. HCl B. $NaC_2H_3O_2$ C. NaCl D. $HC_2H_3O_2$

29. An apple green flame test indicates the presence of

    A. chromium B. sodium C. strontium D. barium

30. In the balanced chemical equation for the reaction between copper and dilute nitric acid, the coefficient before the nitric acid is

    A. 1 B. 3 C. 4 D. 8

31. The molecular weight of sodium hydroxide is 40.
    To prepare 100 cc. of a 0.1 N solution would require a weight of sodium hydroxide, in grams, of

    A. 0.4 B. 2 C. 4 D. 400

32. Concentrated solutions of potassium hydroxide should be stored in bottles with stoppers made of

    A. glass B. rubber C. cork D. aluminum

33. White phosphorus should be stored under

    A. carbon disulfide B. carbon tetrachloride
    C. oil D. water

34. It is dangerous to add concentrated sulfuric acid to

    A. calcium sulfate B. sodium bisulfate
    C. potassium permanganate D. clay

35. You should instruct students to carry concentrated sulfuric acid

    A. very carefully
    B. in a covered metal can
    C. under no circumstances
    D. in a cart

36. The formula for chloroform is

    A. CH_2Cl_2
    B. $CHCl_3$
    C. CH_3Cl
    D. $C_2H_4Cl_2$

37. *Wood* alcohol is the common name for

    A. ethyl alcohol
    B. propyl alcohol
    C. glycerol
    D. methyl alcohol

38. The FIRST thing to do if concentrated acid comes into contact with the skin is to

    A. wash with ammonia
    B. call a doctor
    C. pour sodium hydroxide over it
    D. wash with cold water for a long time

39. Hydrofluoric acid is GENERALLY stored in

    A. polyethylene bottles
    B. glass bottles
    C. copper jars
    D. platinum bottles

40. A liter is APPROXIMATELY equivalent to a(n)

    A. quart
    B. pint
    C. gallon
    D. gill

41. The FIRST scientist to effect a nuclear reaction was

    A. Rutherford
    B. J.J. Thomson
    C. Chadwick
    D. Fermi

42. The chemical behavior of the atom is LARGELY determined by the

    A. atomic weight
    B. number of neutrons
    C. kind of charge in the nucleus
    D. electrons

43. Radioactive substances

    A. easily lose their orbital electrons
    B. have unstable nuclei
    C. gain electrons easily
    D. lack mesons

44. In the reaction $_7N^{15} + {_1H^2} \rightarrow X + {_1H^1}$, X is

    A. $_9F^{17}$
    B. $_8O^{15}$
    C. $_8C^{14}$
    D. $_7N^{16}$

45. In the reaction $C + O_2 \rightarrow CO_2$, the weight of CO_2, in grams, produced by burning 100 grams of carbon with 100 grams of oxygen is about (At. Wgts.: C = 12, O = 16)

    A. 100
    B. 137
    C. 150
    D. 200

46. When sodium combines with chlorine, the sodium is

    A. oxidized and the chlorine is reduced
    B. reduced and the chlorine is oxidized
    C. oxidized and the chlorine remains unchanged
    D. unchanged while the chlorine is oxidized

47. An electric spark is passed through a mixture containing 3.2 grams of oxygen gas and 0.6 grams of hydrogen gas. After the explosion and subsequent cooling to room temperature, there are in the container

    A. 3.2 grams of water and 0.6 grams of hydrogen
    B. 3.6 grams of water and 0.2 grams of hydrogen
    C. 3.8 grams of water and 0 grams of hydrogen
    D. 0.9 grams of water and 2.9 grams of oxygen

48. The columns of the modern periodic table contain elements which resemble each other in

    A. the number of neutrons   B. valence
    C. density   D. appearance

49. Carbon forms a large number of compounds because

    A. of the ability of carbon atoms to form covalent linkages with each other
    B. of its small ionic radius
    C. it forms triple bonds
    D. it is very active

50. The SIMPLEST way to recover silver from a solution of one of its compounds is to

    A. distill the solution   B. use the thermit process
    C. add powdered zinc   D. decompose the solution

KEY (CORRECT ANSWERS)

1. D	11. B	21. C	31. A	41. A
2. C	12. A	22. B	32. B	42. D
3. B	13. C	23. B	33. D	43. B
4. C	14. B	24. D	34. C	44. D
5. A	15. D	25. A	35. C	45. B
6. B	16. A	26. B	36. B	46. A
7. D	17. A	27. B	37. D	47. B
8. D	18. C	28. B	38. D	48. B
9. C	19. A	29. D	39. A	49. A
10. D	20. A	30. D	40. A	50. C

TEST 3

DIRECTIONS: Each question or incomplete statement is followed by several suggested answers or completions. Select the one that BEST answers the question or completes the statement. *PRINT THE LETTER OF THE CORRECT ANSWER IN THE SPACE AT THE RIGHT.*

1. In a chemical reaction, the valence of the element arsenic was changed from +5 to 0. All of the following statements are true EXCEPT the one stating that arsenic   1.____

   A. oxidized something else
   B. was reduced
   C. gained electrons
   D. lost protons

2. The neutralization of a base by an acid ALWAYS produces   2.____

   A. soluble products
   B. water
   C. gas
   D. sodium chloride

3. The pH of an acid solution could be   3.____

   A. 5   B. 7   C. 9   D. 13

4. The CORRECT formula of the hydronium ion is   4.____

   A. OH^- B. H_3O^+ C. H_4O^+ D. H^+

5. When $CaCO_3$ reacts with CHl, the products are   5.____

   A. CaO, H_2O and CO_2
   B. $CaCl_2$, H_2O and CO_2
   C. $CaOCl$, H_2O and CO_2
   D. $CaCl_2$, Cl_2, CO_2 and H_2O

6. A solution of a non-volatile solute in water   6.____

   A. boils at 100° C
   B. freezes below 0° C
   C. has a higher vapor pressure than water at the same temperature
   D. always has a volume equal to the combined volumes of solute and solvent

7. An unknown gas has a density of 1.5 grams per liter under standard conditions. Its molecular weight is about   7.____

   A. 33.6   B. 22.4   C. 11.2   D. 67.2

8. Of the following sequences, the one that CORRECTLY represents the non-metals in the order of their increasing activity as non-metals is   8.____

   A. F, Cl, Br, I
   B. F, I, Cl, Br
   C. I, Cl, Br, F
   D. I, Br, Cl, F

9. Carbon will NOT reduce the oxide of   9.____

   A. sodium   B. iron   C. zinc   D. copper

10. The valence of the metal in the compound $Ca_3(PO_4)_2$ is plus   10.____

    A. 1   B. 2   C. 3   D. 6

11. Covalent bonds are MOST commonly found in

    A. salts
    B. bases
    C. inorganic solids
    D. organic compounds

12. Al_2O_3 and CBr_4, are the correct formulae of the oxide of aluminum and the bromide of carbon.
    The formula of the compound aluminum carbide is

    A. AlC
    B. Al_4C_3
    C. Al_3C_4
    D. Al_4C_2

13. A chalk and salt mixture could be separated into its components by

    A. subliming the salt out of the mixture
    B. adding water and distilling
    C. adding water, boiling, and filtering
    D. adding water, boiling, and cooling

14. The electrolysis of brine is used commercially to produce all of the following substances EXCEPT

    A. sodium hydroxide
    B. hydrogen
    C. chlorine
    D. sodium chloride

15. In the Hall process, cryolite is used as a

    A. source of aluminum
    B. solvent
    C. source of fluorine
    D. solute

16. All of the following are present in pig iron as impurities EXCEPT

    A. silicon
    B. phosphorus
    C. molybdenum
    D. sulfur

17. The compound MOST generally found in petroleum is

    A. $CHCl_3$
    B. C_8H_{18}
    C. CH_5N
    D. $C_7H_{15}OH$

18. When a non-metallic oxide such as N_2O_5 is dissolved in water,

    A. the solution is acidic
    B. the solution is basic
    C. the solution may be either acidic or basic
    D. no chemical change occurs

19. In developing a photographic plate,

    A. sodium thiosulfate is used as a reducing agent
    B. it is left in the developer until all of the silver bromide has been developed
    C. no visible change takes place
    D. the exposed plate is reduced most rapidly where most light has been absorbed

20. The plastic lucite is a polymer of

    A. methyl methacrylate
    B. styrene
    C. butadiene
    D. acrylonitrile

21. MOST animal fats are classed as 21.____

    A. alcohols   B. esters   C. aldehydes   D. acids

22. Hydrogen should be prepared in the classroom by combining 22.____

    A. sodium and hydrochloric acid
    B. zinc and sulfuric acid
    C. potassium chlorate and hydrochloric acid
    D. iron oxide and steam

23. The formula for baking soda is 23.____

    A. Na_2CO_3 B. NaOH   C. $NaHCO_3$ D. Na_2SO_4

24. The chemist GENERALLY credited with discovering deuterium is 24.____

    A. Hall   B. Urey
    C. Fermi   D. Oppenheimer

25. Thermit mixture is composed of 25.____

    A. magnesium and iron oxide
    B. iron and aluminum oxide
    C. aluminum and iron oxide
    D. magnesium and barium peroxide

26. The statement, *It is easier to raise a load with pulleys,* means that for the given load, there is a reduction in the required 26.____

    A. force   B. work   C. distance   D. power

27. If, when three forces are applied to a body, the body is at rest, the resultant of these forces is 27.____

    A. the weight of the object
    B. more than the largest force
    C. zero
    D. the equilibrant of the object

28. Reducing friction has no effect on the 28.____

    A. actual mechanical advantage
    B. efficiency
    C. ideal mechanical advantage
    D. work input

29. Machines can multiply 29.____

    A. work   B. energy   C. force   D. efficiency

30. Weights of 3 lb. and 7 lb. hang from a bar which is supported by a spring scale. Neglecting the weight of the bar, the weight, in pounds, registered by the scale is 30.____

    A. 2.5   B. 4   C. 10   D. 21

31. A body starts from rest and falls freely for four seconds. The distance, in feet, the body will fall (neglecting air resistance) is

    A. 64 B. 96 C. 256 D. 512

32. The width of the film, in inches, used in a 35 mm camera is

    A. 1 B. 1.4 C. 2.5 D. 3.5

33. The pressure cooker cooks food more rapidly because the

    A. water boils more rapidly
    B. water boils at a higher temperature
    C. less water is used
    D. pressure is reduced below normal

34. Any two objects of equal weight are necessarily at the same temperature if

    A. they contain equal amounts of heat
    B. they lose heat at equal rates
    C. neither loses heat to the other when they are in contact
    D. their molecules have equal average speeds

35. Heat may be measured by

    A. temperature change in a known quantity of water
    B. the expansion of mercury
    C. the bending of a bimetallic strip
    D. the expansion of hydrogen

36. The quantity of heat, in calories, required to change 10 grams of ice at 0° C to water at 20° C is

    A. 100 B. 200 C. 1000 D. 5600

37. To double the pressure in a fixed volume of a gas at 0° C, its temperature, in ° C, must be raised to

    A. 100 B. 273 C. 373 D. 546

38. An object is placed 8 inches from a convex lens of 4 inch focal length. The image formed will be

    A. larger than the object
    B. smaller than the object
    C. the same size as the object
    D. virtual

39. When light strikes the prisms in binoculars, it will be

    A. reflected   B. refracted
    C. dispersed   D. absorbed

40. Evidence that light is a transverse wave phenomenon is obtained from

    A. beats   B. polarization
    C. photoelectric effect   D. interference

41. The failure of a lens to focus, at a point, light of different colors is called   41._____

    A. interference   B. spherical aberration
    C. polarization   D. chromatic aberration

42. Two sounds of the same wavelength MUST have the same   42._____

    A. amplitude   B. frequency   C. intensity   D. quality

43. The human ear cannot distinguish tones that differ in   43._____

    A. phase   B. quality   C. intensity   D. pitch

44. Of the following, the one that is at MAXIMUM when resonance occurs in an electrical circuit is   44._____

    A. impedance   B. resistance   C. reactance   D. current

45. Electromagnetic waves radiated into space are called _____ waves.   45._____

    A. rectified   B. carrier
    C. stationary   D. polarized

46. A TV broadcasting station transmits the picture (video signal) by means of _____ modulation of _____ frequency waves.   46._____

    A. frequency; high   B. amplitude; high
    C. frequency; low   D. amplitude; low

47. The emission of electrons from certain metals when they are exposed to light is known as the _____ effect.   47._____

    A. thermionic   B. Edison
    C. photoelectric   D. thermoelectric

48. The process of varying the amplitude of a carrier wave is called   48._____

    A. modulation   B. regeneration
    C. oscillation   D. rectification

49. A transformer may be used to increase   49._____

    A. energy   B. power   C. voltage   D. wattage

50. An induction coil   50._____

    A. produces a large current
    B. changes AC to DC
    C. produces a high voltage
    D. steps down high voltages

KEY (CORRECT ANSWERS)

1. D	11. D	21. B	31. C	41. D
2. B	12. B	22. B	32. B	42. B
3. A	13. C	23. C	33. B	43. A
4. B	14. D	24. B	34. C	44. C
5. B	15. B	25. C	35. A	45. B
6. B	16. C	26. A	36. C	46. B
7. A	17. B	27. C	37. B	47. C
8. D	18. A	28. C	38. C	48. A
9. A	19. D	29. C	39. A	49. C
10. B	20. A	30. C	40. B	50. C

TEST 4

DIRECTIONS: Each question or incomplete statement is followed by several suggested answers or completions. Select the one that BEST answers the question or completes the statement. *PRINT THE LETTER OF THE CORRECT ANSWER IN THE SPACE AT THE RIGHT.*

1. The part NOT found in an AC generator is a(n)   1._____
   - A. field magnet
   - B. armature
   - C. brush(es)
   - D. commutator

2. To protect a delicate watch from a magnetic field, its case should be made of   2._____
   - A. cobalt
   - B. aluminum
   - C. soft iron
   - D. steel

3. The electrical device MOST similar to a galvanometer in operation is the   3._____
   - A. bell
   - B. electromagnet
   - C. motor
   - D. fuse

4. A hand generator is easier to turn when the external circuit is open. This is BEST explained by a principle stated by   4._____
   - A. Oersted
   - B. Ampere
   - C. Ohm
   - D. Lenz

5. *60 cycle* current refers to   5._____
   - A. wavelength
   - B. amplitude
   - C. frequency
   - D. velocity

6. One end of a metal rod is brought near the north pole of a magnet, and it is noted that they attract. This indicates that the metal rod is   6._____
   - A. a permanent magnet
   - B. not a magnet
   - C. a magnetic substance
   - D. made of iron

7. One coulomb per second defines one   7._____
   - A. volt
   - B. watt
   - C. ampere
   - D. ohm

8. Electricity is stored in a   8._____
   - A. dry cell
   - B. condenser
   - C. storage battery
   - D. generator

9. Increasing the distance between the plates of a charged capacitor   9._____
   - A. *increases* the potential difference
   - B. *decreases* the potential difference
   - C. *decreases* the amount of charge
   - D. *increases* the amount of charge

10. A radioactive emission not bent by a magnetic field is a(n)   10._____
    - A. proton
    - B. gamma ray
    - C. beta particle
    - D. alpha particle

11. $_4Be^9$ means that the number of protons in a beryllium nucleus is 11.____

   A. 4   B. 5   C. 9   D. 13

12. *Isotopes* is the name given to elements that have 12.____

   A. the same atomic number but different atomic mass
   B. the same atomic mass but different atomic number
   C. the same atomic mass and the same atomic number but different chemical properties
   D. similar chemical properties although they differ in both atomic mass and atomic number

13. Ionization is the basis for the 13.____

   A. Geiger counter and scintillation counter
   B. Geiger counter and cloud chamber
   C. cloud chamber and scintillation counter
   D. Geiger counter, cloud chamber, and scintillation counter

14. Atomic mass is determined by 14.____

   A. protons   B. neutrons
   C. protons plus neutrons   D. protons minus neutrons

15. The mass of a nucleus, as compared with the sum of the masses of the particles which compose it, is 15.____

   A. slightly greater   B. much greater
   C. equal   D. slightly less

16. To an observer on Earth, the BRIGHTEST planet is 16.____

   A. Jupiter   B. Saturn   C. Mars   D. Venus

17. The Russian Lunik revolves around the 17.____

   A. sun outside the earth's orbit
   B. sun inside the earth's orbit
   C. moon
   D. earth

18. The Northern Cross lies in the constellation 18.____

   A. Cygnus   B. Bootes   C. Lyra   D. Pegasus

19. A galaxy visible to the unaided eye lies in the constellation 19.____

   A. Andromeda   B. Ursa Minor
   C. Auriga   D. Canis Major

20. A rock composed of angular fragments cemented together into a coherent mass is a 20.____

   A. breccia   B. tufa   C. conglomerate   D. dacite

21. In Moh's scale of mineral hardness, quartz is number 21.____

   A. 5   B. 6   C. 7   D. 8

22. A rock which shows foliated structure is

    A. marble   B. serpentine   C. schist   D. quartzite

23. A river is classified as mature when it includes a

    A. chain of lakes in its course
    B. gorge
    C. series of meanders
    D. series of rapids

24. On a Mercator projection, a straight line joining New York City and Liverpool

    A. has constant direction
    B. has constant scale
    C. is the arc of a great circle
    D. has a larger scale near Liverpool than near New York

25. An esker is a

    A. winding, roughly stratified glacial ridge
    B. linear, unstratified glacial ridge
    C. roughly circular glacial mound
    D. series of glacial elevations and depressions

26. An example of an active volcano of the *quiet* type is

    A. Krakatoa   B. Mauna Loa
    C. Mt. Lassen   D. Mt. Vesuvius

27. Stone Mt., Georgia is classified as a

    A. butte   B. mesa
    C. monadnock   D. volcanic neck

28. The velocity of escape of a projectile from the Earth, in number of miles per hour, is about

    A. 7,000   B. 18,000   C. 25,000   D. 35,000

29. An outstanding example of a glacial trough is the

    A. Grand Canyon of the Colorado
    B. Yellowstone Canyon in Yellowstone National Park
    C. Yosemite Valley in Yosemite National Park
    D. Zion Canyon in Zion National Park

30. The Keewatin Glacier of the Pleistocene ice age was centered in

    A. north central Canada   B. Labrador
    C. Alaska   D. Greenland

31. Lost rivers or underground streams are MOST likely to occur in regions whose bedrock is

    A. limestone   B. slate
    C. granite   D. conglomerate

32. The Royal Gorge of the Arkansas River represents a river valley which is

    A. young   B. mature   C. old   D. subdued

33. Sink holes are the result of the work of

    A. earthquakes   B. underground water
    C. streams   D. glaciers

34. The mineral which is LEAST susceptible to chemical weathering is

    A. feldspar   B. hornblends
    C. augite   D. quartz

35. Of the following, the mountains of GREATEST geologic age are the

    A. Appalachians   B. Rockies
    C. Sierra Nevadas   D. Cascades

36. Laccoliths are found in

    A. domed mountains   B. block mountains
    C. folded mountains   D. volcanoes

37. The normal percentage of dissolved mineral matter in sea water (by weight) is APPROXIMATELY

    A. 1.5   B. 2.5   C. 3.5   D. 4.5

38. A shoreline formed as a result of submergence is a _____ shoreline.

    A. coastal plain   B. delta
    C. fiord   D. volcano

39. Spring tides occur at

    A. full moon *only*
    B. new moon *only*
    C. both full and new moon
    D. first and last quarter phases

40. An annular eclipse of the sun takes place at the phase of the moon called

    A. new moon   B. new gibbous
    C. new crescent   D. full moon

41. When it is noon, Eastern Standard Time, in New York City, the standard time at the 120W meridian is

    A. 9 A.M.   B. 10 A.M.   C. 2 P.M.   D. 3 P.M.

42. On June 21, in New York City, the sun

    A. rises in the northeast
    B. sets in the southwest
    C. reaches the zenith at local noon
    D. is north of the zenith at local noon

43. The Palisades of New Jersey originated as an igneous intrusion during the period known as

    A. Eocene
    B. Cretaceous
    C. Permian
    D. Triassic

44. A region whose warmest monthly temperature average is 80° F, while its coldest monthly temperature average is 77° F, MUST have a climate typified as

    A. marine west coast
    B. Mediterranean
    C. tropical desert
    D. tropical rainforest

45. A necessary condition for the formation of sleet is a

    A. cold front
    B. strong pressure gradient
    C. steep lapse rate
    D. temperature inversion

46. The dry adiabatic lapse rate per 1000 feet is

    A. 2.5° F
    B. 3.5° F
    C. 4.5° F
    D. 5.5° F

47. The prevailing wind at 40S latitude is

    A. northwesterly
    B. northeasterly
    C. southwesterly
    D. southeasterly

48. The European equivalent of the American Chinook wind is known as the

    A. bora
    B. buran
    C. foehn
    D. mistral

49. Cumulonimbus clouds are MOST likely to occur in connection with a(n) _____ air mass.

    A. mTk
    B. mTw
    C. cPk
    D. cPw

50. At perigee, our moon's distance, expressed in miles, from the earth is about

    A. 205,000
    B. 220,000
    C. 235,000
    D. 245,000

KEY (CORRECT ANSWERS)

1. D	11. A	21. C	31. A	41. A
2. C	12. A	22. C	32. A	42. A
3. C	13. B	23. D	33. B	43. D
4. D	14. C	24. A	34. D	44. D
5. C	15. D	25. A	35. A	45. D
6. C	16. D	26. B	36. A	46. D
7. C	17. A	27. C	37. C	47. A
8. B	18. A	28. C	38. C	48. C
9. A	19. A	29. C	39. C	49. A
10. B	20. A	30. A	40. A	50. B

EXAMINATION SECTION
TEST 1

DIRECTIONS: Each question or incomplete statement is followed by several suggested answers or completions. Select the one that BEST answers the question or completes the statement. *PRINT THE LETTER OF THE CORRECT ANSWER IN THE SPACE AT THE RIGHT.*

1. Dry ice is

    A. solid carbon dioxide
    B. supercooled water
    C. dehydrated ice
    D. solid air

2. Current concern with population problems has revived interest in the theories of

    A. Darwin   B. DeVries   C. Lamarck   D. Malthus

3. A piece of wood with a specific gravity of 1.1 will

    A. sink
    B. float at the surface
    C. float with 0.1 of its volume above water
    D. float with 0.99 of its volume submerged

4. Isotopes of elements have the same

    A. atomic weight
    B. external system of electrons
    C. number of neutrons in the nucleus
    D. number of electrons and neutrons in the nucleus

5. Sound vibrations are transmitted most rapidly by

    A. steel   B. water   C. air   D. vacuum

6. Graphite and diamond are allotropic forms of

    A. boron   B. cadmium   C. calcium   D. carbon

7. The image on a kineoscope of a television set is formed by a moving beam of light. We see it as a whole picture and as a moving picture because

    A. images persist on the retina
    B. electrons make a fluorescent screen glow
    C. radiant energy stimulates the retina
    D. electrical energy is changed into light energy

8. A large crater discovered in northern Canada not long ago was produced, most likely, by the

    A. explosion of a bomb
    B. eruption of a subterranean volcano
    C. pot-hole erosion of a glacier
    D. impact of a meteorite

9. The fuel best adapted for present day jet airplanes is

    A. naphtha B. gasoline
    C. kerosene D. benzol

10. Which pair is INCORRECTLY matched?

    A. Brass - compound
    B. Sea water - solution
    C. Air - mixture
    D. Milk - emulsion

11. If we compare the eye with a camera, the INCORRECTLY matched pair is

    A. retina - film B. cornea - lens
    C. eyelid - lens cap D. iris - diaphragm

12. Which one of these is NOT a member of the vitamin B complex?

    A. Niacin B. Thiamin C. Lecithin D. Riboflavin

13. A theory to account for the enormous output of solar heat assumes the source to be

    A. the splitting of hydrogen atoms
    B. the destruction of matter during the synthesis of helium
    C. the breakdown of uranium to barium and krypton
    D. loss of neutrons from the sun's interior

14. A metal about to be produced in quantity to aid in the building of jet engines is

    A. gallium B. osmium C. cesium D. titanium

15. Scientists have learned the chemical elements in the sun through the use of the

    A. colorimeter B. spectroscope
    C. telescope D. thermocouple

16. $E = mc^2$. This formula expresses a relationship between energy, mass, and light. It was formulated by

    A. Michaelson B. Bohr
    C. Planck D. Einstein

17. The BEST way to rid a lawn of broadleaf weeds is to

    A. cut the grass very close to the ground
    B. spray with 2, 4-D
    C. inject DDT into the soil
    D. remove each weed individually with a hand spade

18. Glass wool is a good insulator primarily because it

    A. is light in weight
    B. includes many air spaces
    C. is non-inflammable
    D. is relatively inexpensive

19. The term COLD FRONT on a weather map refers to

    A. the region included by isotherms
    B. a region having frosts
    C. an advancing mass of cold air
    D. a region where storms originate

20. Atomic reactors are located on streams. This is necessary in order to

    A. dispose easily of waste products
    B. cool the reactor
    C. facilitate the transportation of needed materials
    D. absorb the radiations in water

21. When a weather report notes nimbus clouds, we may expect

    A. clear weather   B. cold
    C. high winds   D. rain

22. A pigeon whose cerebellum has been removed cannot

    A. breathe   B. swallow food
    C. coordinate its movements   D. see its food

23. The yield of gasoline from crude petroleum is increased by

    A. cracking and hydrogenation
    B. distillation and cracking
    C. distillation and emulsification
    D. hydrogenation and emulsification

24. An effective aid in curing pernicious anemia is

    A. niacin   B. histamine
    C. chloromycetin   D. vitamin B12

25. An electric iron on a 110 volt circuit uses 6 amperes of current. How many kilowatt hours of electricity would it use in 5 hours of ironing?

    A. 33   B. 3.3   C. 330   D. 3300

KEY (CORRECT ANSWERS)

1.	A	11.	B
2.	D	12.	C
3.	A	13.	B
4.	B	14.	D
5.	A	15.	B
6.	D	16.	D
7.	A	17.	B
8.	D	18.	B
9.	C	19.	C
10.	A	20.	B

21. D
22. C
23. A
24. D
25. B

TEST 2

DIRECTIONS: Each question or incomplete statement is followed by several suggested answers or completions. Select the one that BEST answers the question or completes the statement. *PRINT THE LETTER OF THE CORRECT ANSWER IN THE SPACE AT THE RIGHT.*

1. Of the following diseases, the one whose causative agent is of a different type from those of the other three is   1.____

    A. diphtheria
    B. tetanus
    C. poliomyelitis
    D. typhoid fever

2. "Do not move the patient" is a first-aid precept which is applicable particularly in cases of   2.____

    A. bleeding and fainting
    B. fracture and shock
    C. sunstroke and asphyxia
    D. burns and heat exhaustion

3. All of the following statements pertaining to items found in home medicine cabinets are correct EXCEPT: 3.____

    A. Tincture of iodine is unaffected by long storage and hence may be used indefinitely
    B. Hydrogen peroxide is usable as long as it bubbles energetically
    C. Age does not make sedatives dangerous, but they may lose some of their potency with time
    D. If the supply of bicarbonate of soda is exhausted, baking soda may be substituted

4. Of the following, the INCORRECT association of a disease with the period of time during which it is usually communicable is   4.____

    A. impetigo - as long as the sores are unhealed
    B. measles - during the period of running eyes and nose
    C. diphtheria - usually two weeks from the onset of the infection
    D. tetanus - from the onset of the disease to one week later

5. The group of terms which is CORRECTLY arranged in the order of increasing inclusiveness, the least inclusive being stated first, is   5.____

    A. tissues, cells, systems, organs
    B. cells, organs, tissues, organisms
    C. cells, genes, organs, tissues
    D. cells, tissues, organs, systems

6. Ascorbic acid is a vitamin whose presence in foods prevents the occurrence of   6.____

    A. beriberi
    B. night blindness
    C. scurvy
    D. rickets

7. Vitamin A deficiency is associated with all of the following EXCEPT   7.____

    A. faulty development of the teeth
    B. impairment of vision in dim light

C. unhealthy condition of the skin and mucous membranes
D. retardation of the development of bones

8. Aureomycin was developed by

   A. Fleming   B. Banting   C. Waksman   D. Duggar

9. The artificial earth satellites that were planned during the International Geophysical Year by the United States circled the earth in approximately

   A. 1 1/2 hours   B. 1 1/2 days
   C. 1 1/2 weeks   D. 1 1/2 months

10. A class of engines that are NOT of the internal combustion type is

    A. diesel engines   B. gasoline engines
    C. turbo-jet engines   D. steam engines

11. The lead storage battery commonly used in American automobiles is filled with a solution of

    A. sulfuric acid   B. nitric acid
    C. phosphoric acid   D. hydrochloric acid

12. All stars visible to the naked eye belong to

    A. the solar system
    B. a number of galaxies
    C. the Milky Way galaxy
    D. the Milky Way galaxy and several spiral nebulae

13. A poisonous snake native to the eastern United States is the

    A. puff adder   B. king snake
    C. milk snake   D. water moccasin

14. When an observer hears thunder 10 seconds after he sees the lightning flash that caused it, the distance between him and the point of origin of the flash is approximately

    A. 1 mile   B. 2 miles   C. 5 miles   D. 10 miles

15. Rivers flowing into a lake may eventually destroy it by

    A. erosion   B. stream piracy
    C. deposition   D. solution

16. The metal used for the filament of the modern incandescent lamp is

    A. tungsten   B. tantalum   C. thorium   D. titanium

17. The approximate number of miles per degree of latitude of the earth is

    A. 90
    B. 70
    C. 15
    D. widely variable, depending on location

18. The bedrock of a large part of Manhattan is the rock called

    A. granite   B. quartzite
    C. schist   D. trap

19. The function of the cadmium rods in a nuclear reactor is to

    A. slow down neutrons   B. absorb neutrons
    C. speed up neutrons   D. create neutrons

20. The brightest star visible in the night time in New York City is

    A. Betelgeuse   B. Orion
    C. Polaris   D. Sirius

21. A dry cleaning fluid which is not flammable is

    A. carbon disulfide   B. carbon tetrachloride
    C. dimethyl phthalate   D. freon

22. The purpose of making a simple anemometer for a primary grade science lesson is to develop the concept that

    A. air takes up space
    B. the wind blows from different directions
    C. strong winds can destroy things
    D. the wind blows with different amounts of force

23. The normal number of teeth in the adult human being is

    A. 28   B. 32   C. 36   D. 30

24. The reproductive organs of a flowering plant are the

    A. stomata and guard cells
    B. fibrovascular bundles and sieve tubes
    C. pistils and stamens
    D. cambium layer and lenticles

25. A virus is the causative agent of

    A. malaria   B. tetanus
    C. smallpox   D. typhoid fever

KEY (CORRECT ANSWERS)

1.	C	11.	A
2.	B	12.	C
3.	A	13.	D
4.	D	14.	B
5.	D	15.	C
6.	C	16.	A
7.	D	17.	B
8.	D	18.	C
9.	A	19.	B
10.	D	20.	D

21. B
22. D
23. B
24. C
25. C

TEST 3

DIRECTIONS: Each question or incomplete statement is followed by several suggested answers or completions. Select the one that BEST answers the question or completes the statement. *PRINT THE LETTER OF THE CORRECT ANSWER IN THE SPACE AT THE RIGHT.*

1. Which one of the following pairs is INCORRECTLY matched?

    A. Strawberry - eyes
    B. Raspberry - layers
    C. Onion - bulbs
    D. Potato - tubers

2. It was a relatively simple task for Mendel to secure pure lines in the garden pea since in nature it is

    A. wind-pollinated
    B. insect-pollinated
    C. water-pollinated
    D. self-pollinated

3. Respiration in plants

    A. is similar to respiration in animals and takes place at all times
    B. is similar to respiration in animals and takes place only when the plant is not carrying on photosynthesis
    C. is different from respiration in animals and takes place at all times
    D. is different from respiration in animals and takes place only when the plant is not carrying on photosynthesis

4. Modern research indicates that photosynthesis consists

    A. only of rapid light reactions
    B. only of slow light reactions
    C. only of a dark reaction
    D. of a light reaction followed by a dark reaction

5. Cells obtain energy quickly through

    A. photosynthesis
    B. oxidation of glucose
    C. hydrolysis of ATP
    D. osmosis

6. Which one of the following statements with regard to enzymes is NOT true?

    A. Enzymes are organic catalysts produced by living cells.
    B. Enzymes are specific, frequently acting only upon a single substrate.
    C. An enzyme can accelerate a specific reaction in only one direction.
    D. Enzymes have a protein component.

7. A reduction division takes place

    A. only in animal cells during mitosis
    B. only in plant cells during mitosis
    C. in both plant and animal cells during mitosis
    D. in both plant and animal cells during meiosis

8. The essential determiner of heredity in every living cells is a substance known as

    A. DNA
    B. ACTH
    C. 2-4D
    D. ATP

9. If the number of protons in the nucleus of each atom is the same as the number in every other atom, the substance is

    A. inert   B. an active non-metal
    C. amphoteric   D. an element

10. Of the following atomic particles, the lightest in weight is the

    A. proton   B. electron
    C. alpha particle   D. neutron

11. The principal difference between a mixture and a chemical compound is that a

    A. mixture is always heterogeneous in composition
    B. mixture does not contain chemical substances
    C. compound is always of definite composition
    D. compound is more easily separated into its constituent parts

12. Boiling is an effective method of purifying water that contains

    A. soluble organic impurities
    B. bacteria and dissolved gases
    C. insoluble inorganic impurities
    D. soluble organic impurities and bacteria

13. An inexpensive, readily available raw material for the chemical manufacture of washing soda, hydrochloric acid and chlorine is

    A. NaCl   B. Na_2CO_3
    C. HCl   D. $Na_2CO_3 10H_2O$

14. About 75% of the air by weight is

    A. carbon dioxide   B. argon
    C. oxygen   D. nitrogen

15. Argon gas is used to fill tungsten filament electric light bulbs because it

    A. supports the combustion of the filament
    B. offers less resistance to the flow of current than nitrogen
    C. is inert and slows the evaporation of the filament
    D. is less expensive than pure oxygen

16. The number of sub-atomic particles that have been identified is

    A. ten   B. twenty-five
    C. fifty   D. one hundred

17. In ordinary chemical reactions, atoms combine with each other when

    A. electrons are transferred from one atom to the other
    B. nuclear particles are shared
    C. one atom loses protons gained by the other
    D. the transfer of particles produces ions with no electrical charge

18. Adenine, thymine, cytosine, and guanine are all 18._____

    A. chemical names for common vitamins
    B. units that constitute the genetic code of DNA
    C. important hormones
    D. enzymes active in digestion

19. A gas distributed commercially in solid form for use as a refrigerant is 19._____

    A. chlorine   B. carbon dioxide
    C. argon   D. nitrogen

20. Paraffin wax used to make candles is obtained commercially by 20._____

    A. the cracking of kerosene
    B. the dehydrogenation of fuel oil
    C. the fractional distillation of crude oil
    D. polymerization of pure hydrocarbons

21. The E.M.F. that pushes electrons through an electrical circuit is measured in 21._____

    A. ohms   B. volts   C. coulombs   D. amperes

22. The eye abnormality called hyperopic is COMMONLY known as 22._____

    A. astigmatism   B. farsightedness
    C. nearsightedness   D. pink eye

23. The human body is composed MAINLY of which one of the following groups of elements? 23._____

    A. Calcium, phosphorus, iron
    B. Iodine, nitrogen, calcium
    C. Carbon, hydrogen, oxygen
    D. Potassium, oxygen, iron

24. Which one of the following vitamins is NOT a member of the vitamin "B" complex? 24._____

    A. Thiamine   B. Ascorbic acid
    C. Folic acid   D. Niacin

25. Studies indicate that, of the following, the MOST effective procedure for reducing air pollution in cities would be to 25._____

    A. prevent the burning of trash within city limits
    B. use devices to reduce smoke coming from smokestacks
    C. establish controls reducing the discharge of gases from industrial plants
    D. use devices reducing the toxic substances thrown off in the incompletely burned exhausts of automobiles

KEY (CORRECT ANSWERS)

1. A
2. D
3. A
4. D
5. C

6. C
7. D
8. A
9. D
10. B

11. C
12. B
13. A
14. D
15. C

16. D
17. A
18. B
19. B
20. C

21. B
22. B
23. C
24. B
25. D

———

TEST 4

DIRECTIONS: Each question or incomplete statement is followed by several suggested answers or completions. Select the one that BEST answers the question or completes the statement. *PRINT THE LETTER OF THE CORRECT ANSWER IN THE SPACE AT THE RIGHT.*

1. A volt is a unit which measures

   A. electrical pressure
   B. electrical resistance
   C. flow of electricity
   D. volume of electricity

   1.____

2. A room temperature of 68° F is the same as a centigrade temperature of

   A. 34° C   B. 20° C   C. 15° C   D. 42° C

   2.____

3. A calorie is a

   A. substance in food
   B. measure of temperature
   C. substance that produces fat
   D. quantity of heat

   3.____

4. The number of grams equal to one ounce is, approximately,

   A. 2   B. 28   C. 83   D. 12

   4.____

5. A bus comes to a sudden stop. Standing passengers sway forward because of

   A. imbalance
   B. inertia
   C. high center of gravity
   D. centripetal force

   5.____

6. Fanning cools one because it

   A. brings cool air to the surface of the body
   B. blows away warm air
   C. promotes evaporation of perspiration
   D. reduces humidity

   6.____

7. In demonstrating combustion in a small model gas engine, the gasoline becomes ignited. The best extinguisher, of those listed, is

   A. water
   B. an air blower
   C. sawdust
   D. a towel

   7.____

8. Glass wool is a good insulator because it

   A. will not burn
   B. is inexpensive
   C. has many air spaces
   D. is inorganic

   8.____

9. A boy tries to reach for a coin which fell into a pond. He cannot pick it up where it appears to be because of

   A. refraction
   B. reflection
   C. diffraction
   D. diffusion

   9.____

10. Spontaneous generation is an attempted explanation of

   A. the origin of species
   B. how some fires start
   C. birth
   D. origin of living from non-living matter

11. A plant pigment used in the making of starch is

   A. chlorophyl   B. carotin
   C. hemoglobin   D. aniline

12. The sunshine vitamin is

   A. ascorbic acid   B. vitamin A
   C. vitamin D   D. thiamin

13. Pasteurized milk is

   A. milk from inspected cows
   B. milk that has been boiled to kill germs
   C. milk that is free from bacteria
   D. milk that has been heated to a temperature of 145° F

14. In 1892, Newark began to purify its drinking water. This has resulted in a marked reduction in death from

   A. tuberculosis   B. infantile paralysis
   C. typhoid fever   D. malaria

15. Penicillin is a(n)

   A. germicide   B. antibiotic
   C. antiseptic   D. disinfectant

16. A disease of white corpuscles is

   A. pernicious anemia   B. leukemia
   C. malaria   D. phagocytosis

17. Sulfa drugs have been used successfully in treating

   A. cancer   B. rickets
   C. infantile paralysis   D. pneumonia

18. Some animals and plants can live under water because they

   A. do not need oxygen
   B. use dissolved oxygen
   C. decompose water molecules to get oxygen
   D. use water in place of oxygen

19. Some plants can make direct use of nitrogen from the air as a result of the process of

   A. absorption   B. osmosis
   C. infiltration   D. fixation

20. A natural body defense against disease germs is

    A. fresh air B. saliva
    C. white corpuscles D. enzymes

21. Seasons result from

    A. the revolution and the rotation of the earth
    B. the revolution and the inclination of the earth
    C. the variation of the distance of the earth from the sun
    D. the variation in radiation from the sun

22. A mutant is

    A. a plant graft
    B. a dumb person
    C. a hybrid
    D. an organism with a new heritable trait

23. The Dick test is a test for susceptibility to

    A. diphtheria B. scarlet fever
    C. tuberculosis D. virus infection

24. For an average-sized man doing moderately hard physical work, the caloric intake per day should be close to

    A. 6000 calories B. 2000 calories
    C. 3500 calories D. 1200 calories

25. In a balanced diet for an average person, the proportion of carbohydrates, fats, and proteins should be

    A. 2:2:1 B. 3:2:1 C. 3:1:1 D. 1:2:1

KEY (CORRECT ANSWERS)

1.	A	11.	A
2.	B	12.	C
3.	D	13.	D
4.	B	14.	C
5.	B	15.	B
6.	C	16.	B
7.	D	17.	D
8.	C	18.	B
9.	A	19.	D
10.	D	20.	C

21. B
22. D
23. B
24. C
25. C